Dr Mike Smith's Postbag
SKIN PROBLEMS

Dr Mike Smith is a specialist in preventative medicine and a general practitioner. He was the Chief Medical Officer of the Family Planning Association 1970–75 and their Honorary Medical Adviser 1975–90. He is an elected member of the FPA's National Executive Committee, a member of the Pet Health Council and a member of the advisory panel of the National Food Safety Advisory Centre. For many years he has been a 'resident' expert guest on BBC Radio 2's *Jimmy Young Show*, LBC's *Nightline* and the medical columnist/editor for *Woman's Own*. Between 1988 and 1990 he was the expert guest on SKY TV's *Sky by Day*. In April 1991 he was voted the TV and Radio Doctors' 'Expert's Expert' in the *Observer* magazine's series.

As well as the Postbag series, he is also the author of *Birth Control, How to Save Your Child's Life, A New Dictionary of Symptoms, Dr Mike Smith's Handbook of Over-the-Counter Medicines, Dr Mike Smith's Handbook of Prescription Medicines* and *Dr Mike Smith's First Aid Handbook* (to be published May 1994).

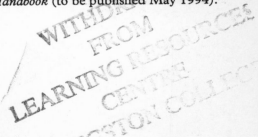

DR MIKE SMITH'S

POSTBAG

SKIN PROBLEMS

WITH SHARRON KERR

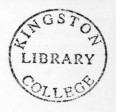

KYLE CATHIE LIMITED

First published in Great Britain in 1994 by
Kyle Cathie Limited
7/8 Hatherley Street, London SW1P 2QT

ISBN 1 85626 122 0

Dr Mike Smith is hereby identified as the author of this
work in accordance with Section 77 of the Copyright, Designs
and Patents Act 1988.

A Cataloguing in Publication record for this title is
available from the British Library.

Typeset by Heronwood Press, Medstead, Hampshire
Printed in Great Britain by Cox and Wyman Ltd, Reading

CONTENTS

INTRODUCTION

Skin problems are many and varied. They all have different causes and require different treatments. And while it may be true that in the main the conditions do not endanger life, they can still cause great distress. After all, if you have high blood pressure, a peptic ulcer, or arthritis even, you can keep that private. People will only know if you want them to know. With a skin problem like eczema or psoriasis it's usually visible to everyone – friend and stranger alike – particularly when the face and hands are affected.

As well as the physical effects of skin problems, such as pain, inflammation or itching, the psychological consequences are enormous. In some instances these effects are far worse than the physical harm. So many sufferers tell me that they believe not enough is written or talked about regarding these psychological aspects. They believe other people fail to understand how sufferers can become angry or depressed, how they can hate or be ashamed of their bodies and how these feelings can complicate or prevent personal relationships.

Sufferers of skin problems often feel a lack of self-worth, partly due to the way they see themselves and partly because of the way they have to cope with other people's reactions to their appearance. One young woman who has suffered from eczema for more than twenty years told me that she truly believed her personality would have been quite different if she had not had a skin problem.

I was bullied and teased as a child because of my eczema. Other children thought that it was contagious. I used to cry a lot and it made me a very insecure person. Now, as a result, I have a tendency to want to please people. I'm a bit over-sensitive and I'm always apologising for things. Even as an adult I feel my skin condition has affected my self-esteem.

Another eczema sufferer once told me how she was filled with self-disgust because of her problem. She was trapped in a cycle of itching then scratching. Unable to stop herself from scratching hard, her skin would bleed and she wouldn't be able to sleep at night. In the morning her skin would have crusted over and she would often find her body sticking to the sheets. She felt disgusted with herself.

THE SKIN

So many of us trivialise the importance of healthy skin. It's not *just* a skin, it's far more than that. Its role is vital and incredibly complex.

The skin is made up of two sections. The epidermis is the outer section, which has four main layers, and the dermis is the lower section, which has two layers. The epidermis is the waterproof layer which protects us against invasion by bacteria. The dermis, among its other functions, acts as a cushion, with a good supply of fat cells which prevent the skin wearing through in those areas, for example, where it is stretched over a bony prominence.

Skin is a pretty tough covering which makes us waterproof and leakproof. It also plays an important part in our body's defences – aside from the physical cover, it produces antibodies against invading germs and other noxious substances (poisons that we may come into contact with every day). This function can over-react should we become sensitised to a substance and further contact with it can produce anything from a rash to a sudden and sometimes dramatic swelling. This can occur with nickel, for example, and with some of the older antibiotics which, as a result, are never used in skin ointments.

We have about two square metres of skin, making it the largest organ in the body, comprising thousands of components including sweat glands, sebaceous glands, blood vessels, nerve endings, sensory cells, heat and cold receptors, touch receptors, hairs and muscles.

Skin has many different functions. For example, it has the main body mechanism for reducing our temperature in a hot environment. With every cc of sweat that evaporates, 540 calories of heat are carried away with it – enough to warm 540 ccs of water to 1°C. We can also excrete certain waste products through the skin via the sweat. In addition, the small blood vessels just under the surface can readily open and close, allowing the body's heat to be conserved in the cold or be given out when we're hot. Our flesh goes red when the vessels open, turning the skin into a natural radiator.

The skin's sebaceous glands give off sexually attractive odours, especially under the arms and in the intimate genital areas. In modern times, however, we have become used to regular baths and the perfume producers' artificial odours, so if left there too long stale sebaceous secretions can also be a turn-off!

In this book I have tried to cover only those skin conditions that the everyday reader will recognise. I give an idea of the causes of these conditions, the symptoms and treatments but, as ever in medicine, there is much that we don't know about why one person should get a condition – psoriasis, for example – while others do not. One suspects that the susceptibility is carried in the genes. As our knowledge of genes is advancing so rapidly perhaps when I update this book we will be more confident about the cause of many of the conditions – and so well on our way to preventing them.

1: ACNE

Acne is a disorder of the sebaceous glands in the skin which causes spots. It's probably one of the most distressing of the common skin conditions and affects almost all youngsters at some time or another. It can vary in severity from just a few spots to being quite disfiguring, although such severe cases are rare. It's one of the few problems that is generally worse in men and it's been shown that if your parents had a problem with spots then you are more likely to suffer than someone whose parents did not.

Spots usually first appear when the sufferer is between the ages of eleven and fifteen, and disappear when he or she is in their mid-twenties. In fact, acne is usually at its worst in girls when they are about seventeen and in boys at around eighteen or nineteen. In rare and depressing cases the spots can continue into the late thirties, even up until forty. This happens in about one in twenty female sufferers and about one in a hundred male sufferers.

Acne affects the skin on the face, neck, back and chest. However the face is the area which tends to be affected the most – and not all sufferers will have spots on their back or chest.

Spots normally occur because of an increase in the production of sebum, the skin's normal oily secretion. Sebum keeps the skin moist and supple – without it, it would become dry and might even crack. Over-production of sebum is due to stimulation from a male hormone, androgen, and leads to the shiny skin common in teenagers. With the increase in this skin grease, the pores can become blocked and infected by bacteria which thrive on the sebum. This in turn causes spots.

Acne spots can be described either as inflamed spots

or non-inflamed spots. Non-inflamed spots are called whiteheads or blackheads; inflamed spots are papules, pustules, nodules or cysts. Blackheads are very small black spots which usually appear around the nose and chin. They are caused by dead skin cells and sebum collecting in a hair follicle and becoming discoloured by exposure to air. Inflamed spots have white centres caused by bacterial activity in sebum which has collected in a hair follicle. In severe cases, nodules or larger cysts develop – tender, swollen lumps under the skin caused by scar tissue forming around an inflamed area.

Acne can lead to scarring, particularly from nodules and cysts, although with the improvements in treatment the risk of being left with a scar has been dramatically reduced. Most cases of acne can now be kept under control until the sufferer reaches an age when it will clear up naturally. The kind of acne most likely to cause scarring is cystic acne, for which the treatment is usually a small, daily dose of antibiotics.

HOW ACNE IS TREATED

Clearing up acne nearly always requires great perseverance. There is no overnight cure and you may have to persist with treatment for several months at a time. What is often forgotten, however, is that the treatment needs to be used constantly – not just to treat a particular outbreak. Sufferers who stop once the spots get better soon find that they return (as in our case study on page 11).

The most common form of treatment available is a keratolytic skin ointment – this 'dissolves' the keratin (top layer of the skin) and encourages peeling of the layer of dead and hardened cells that form the skin's surface. Keratolytics are effective because, like sunlight, they promote skin peeling and in that way help unblock pores and dry up the extra grease. Products available usually contain the keratolytics benzoyl peroxide, sulphur or salicylic acid. Benzoyl peroxide and sulphur also have an anti-bacterial effect. Or you can buy a product called Acnidazil, for example, which combines benzoyl peroxide with an anti-bacterial agent called miconazole.

Keratolytic preparations often cause soreness so are available in different strengths. Benzoyl peroxide, for instance, is likely to cause a mild burning sensation on the first application, as well as a moderate reddening and peeling of the skin during the first few days. Throughout the initial few weeks of treatment, most patients will experience a sudden increase in peeling. This isn't harmful and will subside within a day or two if treatment is temporarily discontinued. Then start treatment again and continue while the acne is kept at bay and the other side-effects remain at non-worrying levels. If discomfort, such as burning, redness or excessive peeling, does occur, stop the treatment temporarily or consult a doctor. Preparations containing benzoyl peroxide shouldn't be used for longer than three months at a time.

It's also worth noting that these products may bleach clothing and fabrics, so use them with care.

These preparations can be obtained on prescription or you can choose from a wide selection of acne treatments in your local pharmacy. As well as keratolytic skin ointments, you'll find a selection of anti-bacterial skin-washing creams, lotions and soaps. These can help by reducing bacterial activity in the skin. Antiseptic creams, ointments and soaps can destroy micro-organisms, and abrasives can remove blockages clogging up the pores. You can also buy homoeopathic treatments in pharmacies and health shops – those said to be good for acne are *Belladonna*, *Hepar. Sulph.*, *Pulsatilla*, *Silicea* and *Sulphur*.

If you have sensitive skin, or have suffered adverse

reactions to other acne preparations in the past, it's worth applying creams or lotions to a small area for the first few days. If your skin seems to tolerate it, you can then treat the larger areas.

If keratolytic ointments or other treatments don't work for you, don't give up hope. And do visit your doctor to seek his or her advice. He or she may recommend a different form of treatment – a lotion, gel or cream containing tretinoin (derived from vitamin A) or one with an antibiotic. There is also an antibiotic/anti-inflammatory topical treatment such as Zineryt, which may cause a slight burning sensation or a slight redness of the skin, due to its alcohol base.

Your doctor may even refer you to a specialist dermatologist, who will possibly prescribe vitamin A derivative capsules such as Roaccutane (isotretinoin). Isotretinoin dramatically reduces the formation of grease by the sebaceous glands, cuts down on the formation of non-inflamed lesions and the amount of bacteria and also reduces inflammation. It's an effective treatment for severe acne but not without side-effects – in particular it can damage an unborn child if taken during pregnancy. So women should be careful not to become pregnant while taking the drug, and should use contraception for at least four weeks before treatment, all the time during it and for at least four weeks after it's stopped (even women with a history of infertility). Most patients experience drying of the lips, skin (particularly on the face) and even eyelids. Up to three in ten develop mild aches and pains of the joints or muscles and 15 per cent suffer headaches.

Vitamin A-derivative capsules can have dramatic results. As I've said, they work by suppressing sebum production – with less grease, bacteria are discouraged, as are blackheads and whiteheads which may go on to develop into larger spots. Unfortunately, these capsules are very expensive which limits the number of NHS patients who can benefit from them.

If you're female the doctor may suggest the use of a contraceptive pill – either a common one which is known also to be beneficial to the skin or one which, while still having a contraceptive effect, is primarily prescribed for the treatment of acne – for example, Dianette.

Antibiotics can, as I said earlier, be prescribed for acne – the most common are tetracycline or oxytetracycline – usually for a period of six months (but remind the doctor if you are on the pill). Other antibiotics include erythromycin, minocycline, doxycycline and trimethoprim. Antibiotics work in two ways – they reduce both the amount of bacteria and the inflammatory response. This type of treatment is normally thought to be very safe, although rarely an itchy rash can occur, in which case treatment should be stopped. Other infrequent side-effects include sickness or abdominal pain, or mild diarrhoea.

SELF-HELP TREATMENT

If you suffer from acne, you should try to avoid worrying about your spots, since that won't make them any better. I know this can be very difficult for sufferers of severe acne. For some the condition can take over their lives, driving them away from people, from crowds, from strangers, even from acquaintances. It would take someone with a very devil-may-care attitude not to let such dreadful acne upset their lives. Dame Edna Everage tells a joke about 'her' daughter's acne being 'terminal'. Well, it can certainly be terminal to a sufferer's pride, self-confidence and social life.

Restrain yourself from squeezing blackheads as this can cause further damage and a scarring of the skin. It can also cause the spots to spread. Many acne sufferers try not to eat chocolate and other fatty foods, and although there is no real proof that this has any effect, it's worth a try, as a healthy, well-balanced diet with plenty of fresh fruit and vegetables can only be good for you. Sunshine can help dry up your spots – but don't overdo it and burn yourself. Sunlight can improve the look of your skin in the short term because it promotes skin peeling, helping to unblock pores and dry up excess grease.

CASE STUDY: MARGARET

About three-quarters of young women with acne find that their spots get worse just before their period. Margaret was no exception. She's twenty-five and has suffered from spots since she was about thirteen, though thankfully her acne has now virtually cleared up.

I don't even clearly remember when spots started to appear on my face. It seems as if I woke up one morning and there they all were. But I'm sure it didn't really happen that way. I do remember that getting spots was yet one more change in my life. And all these changes seemed to be happening at the same time which made me feel quite unsettled and unsure of myself.

First of all there were the physical changes: my body was changing shape, my breasts were developing, I was suddenly growing pubic hair, then my periods started and on top of all that I had a spotty face. I had long hair which was thick and shiny and I had always been proud of that. Now it looked as if someone had poured olive oil all over it. I had to wash it virtually every day. If I didn't, my fringe would almost be sticking to my forehead because of the grease. My face felt very greasy too. I can remember feeling as if I was dirty and unclean all the time and worried that other people would think I hadn't washed. I really did begin to feel that growing up wasn't a very pleasant experience. I can remember one night in my bedroom I just cried for the childhood I was about to surrender, which seems really silly because when I look back it was inevitable after all!

By about the age of sixteen Margaret's spots were probably at their worst. However she was fortunate that

she wasn't teased and didn't feel the odd one out because so many other girls in her year at school had the
same kind of problem.

I wouldn't say that my acne was severe in any way. I think
it was just the run-of-the-mill type. I can remember thinking that there were quite a few of us who had spotty skin.
Although I remember too that there were girls at school
who didn't seem to have spots or greasy hair. I wasn't jeal-
ous of them, but I did feel a bit fed up that it had to be me
who had all the spots, especially as I had to wear a brace as
well.

There were times when the spots were pretty painful.
From what I remember, I seemed to have a variety of different types. Across my forehead there were hundreds of
tiny pimples. I know you weren't supposed to squeeze the
spots or scratch them but that's really hard. I'd be in
lessons and sometimes be concentrating and leaning on my
arm and scraping my fingernails across all the spots, sometimes bursting one or two of them on the way. It sounds
disgusting but it was almost addictive, especially as I had so
many. Once I started it was difficult to stop.

I used to get lots of blackheads around my nose and chin.
And also on my chin I'd get really big spots that would be
full of pus. I used to squeeze those too but I always made
sure I cleaned the area with an antiseptic like TCP before
and after. I also used to get quite a few patches of quite big
pimples on my back. These could be very painful, especially when my clothes rubbed against them or when someone bumped into me or the strap from my bag caught
against them.

It's easy for people to tell you not to squeeze spots but
the yellow pus used to make me feel so embarrassed, and
not only that, the pressure it built up in my skin would
make the spots very painful. Sometimes a spot could really
throb. The most painful type I used to get would look like a
small round lump under the skin. These would hurt so
much but they would never come to a head. They would
take days to heal. Luckily I didn't get those that often.

I used to try all sorts of things to get rid of the spots during the first couple of years, but eventually I just forgot
about them – apart from using an anti-bacterial facewash in

the morning and evening, which seemed to help a bit. I tried all sorts of creams and ointments, more recently ones containing benzoyl peroxide. They used to help a little but I didn't realise then that you needed to use them for quite a long time to really get any benefit. I used to get fed up with applying them after a couple of weeks. I thought that if my spots came back it meant that the creams and ointments weren't working. I didn't realise that I should have kept on with the treatment for much longer than I did. I've since read that I should also have kept on treating my skin when spots had cleared a bit in order to stop them coming back.

I tried homoeopathic medicine, too. I was given these little sachets of powders to take. These seemed to help the acne a bit – most things helped a bit but nothing used to get rid of it completely. I quite enjoyed having homoeopathic treatment because I felt the woman treating me took time to talk to me and to ask me about my life, rather than just scribbling out a prescription in about thirty seconds flat.

I also used to try anything that I read about in teenage magazines, such as face packs, or cutting out chocolate and fatty foods, but that never made much difference to my skin or my greasy hair. Most of the time I used to try to make sure my hair covered my face as much as possible to try to hide all the spots, and I sometimes wonder whether that made them even worse! I did find that going on the pill when I was about eighteen certainly made quite a difference to my skin and the number of spots did reduce quite a lot. I just used to get a few painful spots on my chin but the crop on my forehead went. Now I just seem to get them in the few days before my period.

I was lucky, acne didn't cause me great embarrassment, but I did used to get very upset that my spots always seemed to get worse whenever I wanted to go somewhere special. If we had a school dance you can bet I'd have a face full of spots. There were one or two dances that I didn't even go to because of my skin. I told my friends I had a sore throat. I would never have admitted that I didn't want to go because I thought no one would dance with me with so many spots and grease on my face. My mother used to try to cheer me up by telling me not to worry and that my skin would clear up when I got older. That just used to make me feel even more grumpy – she'd told me so many times and I didn't really believe it anyway. But fortunately for me she was right and my skin is now so much better than it used to be. My hair's not so greasy either!

2: DERMATITIS AND ECZEMA

'What's the difference between dermatitis and eczema?' is a question I'm asked time and again. Well, eczema and dermatitis are used as virtually interchangeable terms and generally mean inflammation of the skin. The word dermatitis is the more general of the two descriptions, as it can be used for *any* inflammation of the skin (the name is derived from Old English – *derma* meaning skin, *itis* meaning inflammation).

Eczema isn't just one skin problem – it's used more as a description of a skin reaction characterised, when seen under the microscope, by water-logging of the top layer of skin – the epidermis. The term eczema is derived from the Greek word *eczein*, which means to boil or bubble over, so the term eczema is really quite descriptive. The main symptoms are itching, redness and swelling, accompanied by small blisters which often weep and form a crust. It's thought that as many as one in ten or even two out of ten people suffer from eczema and it can range in severity quite drastically.

DIFFERENT KINDS OF DERMATITIS AND ECZEMA

Atopic eczema (or infantile eczema)

Atopic eczema is thought to be the result of outside factors combining with a person's inherited tendency to sensitive skin. It's unusual for this type of eczema to develop in adult life and most symptoms begin to appear within the first two years after birth – sometimes as early as six weeks. Initially this type of eczema usually manifests itself on the face, scalp and nappy area and as a child grows it can develop on the neck, hands, feet, arms and legs. About one child in ten suffers from this condition. The symptoms are similar to those described above, but may look worse as a result of the child's scratching. Consult your doctor for treatment and advice.

Parents can often be very concerned that they have 'spread' eczema to their child, that the child has caught it like an infectious disease. I receive many letters from anxious parents about this. A common letter goes something like this, 'I've had eczema in my adult years and now my GP has just diagnosed eczema on my baby's neck and ankles. Could he have caught this condition from me?'

From the details given in the letters, and from what their doctors have told them, I can usually reassure these mums and dads. Their skin condition often sounds like a dermatitis caused by a reaction to something in their home or workplace. Such a dermatitis is more likely to occur for the first time in adults. This kind is not 'caught' like an infectious disease.

The atopic variety definitely runs in families. Sufferers usually have a higher level of one particular antibody in their blood – the E group. It's likely that this is why their skin 'boils' with eczema, particularly when they come into contact with irritants such as certain metals, soaps, detergents and pollens. Some fortunate sufferers may be able to identify eczema triggers and therefore avoid them in the future – but for most people this is difficult to do.

One thing I always say to parents is: whichever type you have, don't blame yourself for your child's condition. Sometimes the eczema genes may skip a generation or two and you may not even be aware of anyone in your family having had a skin problem. Fortunately, for many young atopic sufferers, the symptoms clear up as they reach adult life. Some figures I have read suggest that 90 per cent of children with eczema grow out of it by the age of eight, though in my experience it tends to be later than that – and for some, unfortunately, much later.

Many atopic sufferers might also be allergic to a variety of different things such as pollen and certain foods – eggs, fish, nuts and fruit, for example. Sometimes contact with cats, dogs or other furry animals can trigger eczema and contact with the house-dust mite can play a part, too. These tiny creatures, invisible to the naked eye, exist in their millions in the furnishings, floors and bedding of even the cleanest home. They live on the dead skin cells that we constantly shed and each produces forty faecal pellets a day – not a pretty thought! Fortunately, most of us co-exist quite happily with these mites, but their pellets are often the trigger for an allergic response in the susceptible. The manufacturers of bedding protection now spray or paint on mite protectors, and vacuum cleaner filter producers have played their part in pointing out the potential dangers of the mite.

The role of food allergies in atopic eczema is also cause for debate. It's likely that only a very few sufferers can really be helped by modifying what they eat, though some have found that avoiding dairy products altogether eases the condition. But, should you want to alter your child's diet, especially a child under four, you should always consult your doctor or health visitor first.

It's also thought that breastfeeding may help prevent eczema. Atopic eczema is less common in breastfed babies perhaps because, the milk being the natural food, it is unlikely to contain allergens – the triggers that set off the symptoms.

Contact dermatitis

Another form of skin complaint is known as contact dermatitis. This has similar symptoms to eczema but is specifically caused by contact with substances to which your skin is sensitive or substances which are an irritant to the skin. It's a very common problem. I'm sure many people will have come across some product or substance which has irritated their skin – be it washing powder or other household detergents, or costume jewellery, for example. Something like one in ten British women is allergic to nickel, which is used in frames for glasses, jewellery and metal clothing accessories. Lanolin is another common irritant. This is often used in cosmetics and facial cleansing products, though these days many products are labelled lanolin-free – which is very helpful to sufferers.

It's amazing just how many people contract dermatitis as a result of becoming sensitive to nickel. It can sometimes be difficult to diagnose as the sufferer may have the rash on parts of the body not in direct contact with the metal. While a rash under the trigger article – a ring or a bracelet, for example – may immediately pinpoint the cause, a response elsewhere on the body arises from a different immune mechanism. As a result, one often needs the opinion of a skin specialist to make a firm diagnosis.

When an industrial irritant is responsible, the diagnosis will usually be straightforward. Doctors who specialise in occupational health will be on the lookout for it, having made a study of such trigger substances, and will be very careful to ensure that the industrial processes in question provide sufficient protection. This can be achieved by the use of suitable extractor fans and protective clothing, and by the enclosure of the particular process so that it's no longer able to contaminate the working environment.

A problem for many in the building trade, for example, is wet cement. This can frequently cause contact dermatitis, as Jack, a sixty-four-year-old plumber, discovered. He found that whenever he worked with wet cement, he would have a rash on his hands. He also found that contact with washing up liquid produced a similar rash.

I once had such a bad reaction to wet cement that I had to have six months off work. I had been laying pipes for drains which needed cement joints. I didn't even think that I needed to wear gloves – and anyway, gloves don't really go with a builder's macho image!

The job lasted two weeks. It involved handling cement for about five hours every day. After a few days my hands began to feel quite irritated and the skin was becoming dry. It got worse after a week when little cracks and tiny blisters began to appear all over the back of my hands and particularly between the fingers. At the end of the fortnight my hands were really sore and itchy. In fact, they became so bad that I needed the six months off work while the skin healed and I was able to use my hands properly again.

After that incident I always tried to wear gloves when I had to use cement, macho image or not, and this helped prevent any further episodes. I also found that I had to be careful about washing up and I need to wear rubber gloves. If I don't the washing up liquid causes the skin on my hands to become so dry that it cracks easily and then develops blisters.

If you suffer from contact dermatitis it's important, wherever possible, to avoid contact with the aggravating substance, and any rash should be treated immediately with anti-inflammatory medicines – usually applied as creams, but occasionally taken orally. Once a specific diagnosis has been made, the sufferer often feels much happier in the knowledge that they haven't got some sinister disease, just an over-reaction of the body's defences to a substance which irritates or provokes an allergy.

Seborrhoeic dermatitis

Seborrhoeic dermatitis, or seborrhoea for short, ranges from severe dandruff (see page 66) to a wet eruption of the scalp and other hairy areas of the body, for example, the chest and groin. It can cause the skin to flake off and can be uncomfortably itchy.

In this condition, which is most common in young men but can affect women too, the flakes of skin are large, yellow and oily. The skin on the scalp becomes red, inflamed and soggy, especially around the edges and may be infected by other germs. Eyelashes, eyebrows, skin folds on either side of the nose and behind the ears can all be affected, as can other parts of the body, such as the chest, armpits, breasts and groin.

Dandruff, considered by many doctors to be a very mild form of seborrhoeic dermatitis, can be socially distressing. As many sufferers have told me, a flaking of the scalp can restrict the colour of the clothes you wear. Navy blue, black and other dark colours contrast so markedly with even a few flakes that most sufferers confine themselves to white or very pale colours. Just imagine how sufferers must feel when huge flakes start to descend within moments of putting on an outfit. And when eyebrows, eyelashes and other noticeable areas of the skin become affected, it can be a calamity.

But over the past few years, the outlook has become brighter for sufferers. Previously they had coped the best they could, making do with the traditional coal-tar and other preparations, but there are now new theories about what actually causes seborrhoea. One of the most recent and exciting of these theories is that the sufferer reacts to a yeast-type or fungal germ which is present in the air. A close relative of yeast, known as a dermatophyte, covers all of our skin, but only the seborrhoeic dermatitis or dandruff sufferer seems to react to its presence.

So new treatments aimed at eliminating this dermatophyte – either by destroying it, or by seeing that it doesn't feed – could be the way to overcome this long-standing problem.

A prescribed anti-fungal shampoo can work absolute

wonders, since the fungus – which floats in the air and lands on us all the time – can't be avoided (see page 67). Doctors will recommend these shampoos to treat dermatophytes that affect the skin on other parts of the body, but of course they won't do this until they've made a firm diagnosis that it is a dermatophyte or similar germ which is responsible.

Seborrhoeic eczema

This is a similar type of eczema affecting young babies, which often appears between six weeks and three months. It looks like a bad case of nappy rash and the scalp is also affected. Thick, yellow scales develop on the scalp and they can extend on to the forehead and below. Mild forms of this are generally known by the more common name of 'cradle cap' (see page 67). The good news is that this can often disappear by the time the baby is a year old.

As with seborrhoeic dermatitis, the condition is provoked by an unseen fungus so you can treat it with antifungal creams or shampoos.

Discoid eczema

This is also referred to as nummular eczema and involves circular patches of dry, red skin on the limbs and trunk, caused by a drying out of the skin. Often simple moisturizing bath additives or creams will be all that's needed once the diagnosis is made. This form is not as common as the other types of eczema.

The condition mostly tends to occur in people over fifty who live in centrally heated houses. This is because the warm air inside a heated house can 'hold' more moisture than the colder air outside. Consequently, warm air inside the house readily absorbs moisture from our skin – and also the furniture! In the alps, for example, where the very cold air outside delivers very dry air into a centrally heated chalet, the wooden furniture can almost curl with dryness unless electric vaporisers are used to increase the moisture (known as the 'relative humidity') of the inside air.

Varicose eczema

Chronic venous hypertension in the lower leg can cause varicose eczema, also called stasis dermatitis. Hypertension means that the pressure within the veins is higher than nature intended, and 'stasis' means that the blood is moving far slower than it should – it 'complains' by producing the distressing eczema rash, especially common on the inside of the ankle (nobody knows why). This can be quite problematic because here the skin is often less resilient and could ulcerate. This is one reason why varicose veins should not be ignored. They can be treated either by injection, to shrivel them up, or by an operation to tie them off and remove them. They can, at least, be relieved by supporting the tissues of the leg with carefully fitted graduated support stockings or tights.

Eczema craquele

Also called asteatotic eczema, this is a kind of eczema that generally affects older people. The skin, especially on the lower legs, can become dry and itchy, looking not unlike crazy paving. As we get older the rate of sebum begins to decrease, causing the skin to become dry and cracked.

This problem can often develop as a result of a hospital stay, as the warm environment together with strict hygiene rules and regular washing can lead to overdryness of the skin.

Although this is a problem common in the elderly, reports suggest that more and more older people are suffering from eczema in general. One likely explanation is that there are now more pollutants in the atmosphere and home than ever before.

As often as not, the treatment depends on keeping the skin as moisturised as possible, either with bath, cream or ointment moisturising preparations.

One thing is definite though, no matter what your age, when you develop a skin problem for the first time you should consult your GP.

Neurodermatitis

This is sometimes called dermatitis artefacta. It's often a small patch of skin that we habitually scratch without even thinking about it, usually at times of anxiety. One of the Eczema Society leaflets describes it rather poetically as the 'worry beads' of our skin. Quite often on the face, it becomes a sore spot that is usually red due to the inflammation caused by the constant scratching. It almost always has a crust or a scab where the rubbed away skin is unable to heal because it is continually disturbed. Over the years, if the scratching continues, it quite often loses its pigment and appears white at the centre.

Pompholyx

This appears as small blisters on the soles of the feet or palms of the hands, and can be very itchy. It may also be referred to as vesicular or dishydrotic eczema. However it's not really a specific type of eczema rather a complication of it.

TREATMENT

Eczema can take the form of small red patches on the limbs or it can afflict large areas of the body – it is very unpredictable. When it finally does calm down, there is no guarantee it won't return later as bad as ever. Someone who's had eczema for a very long time may even find that areas of their skin become thickened.

The degree to which the skin is dry, flaky, hot and itchy depends on the severity of the attack; in very bad cases it will be broken, sensitive, raw and bleeding. Life can become intolerable and for some a hospital stay is the only option.

Although it is not usually considered a 'serious disease', it can still be severe, uncomfortable and unsightly, causing much self-consciousness. Eczema is not contagious, yet its unsightly appearance can make other people wary, causing the sufferer to feel embarrassed, distressed or isolated. For some this lack of confidence can be more difficult to cope with than the eczema itself.

There are many misconceptions regarding eczema, and children are often cruelly teased by their peers about their skin. As with so many other similar and chronic conditions – the wheezing of asthma, for instance – this is most unfair. People can't help having their condition and deserve our sympathy, not our taunts.

If you think you have eczema, see your doctor. Although it is often hard to define the cause of the problem or to cure it completely, there are a number of treatments available that will control it – emollients that moisturise the skin, anti-pruritics, topical steroids, antifungals, antibiotics and antihistamines. However, you must bear in mind that although the eczema may clear up, the skin will probably always remain sensitive.

Steroids

Steroids are near-relatives of many of the natural hormones produced in our body – for instance, secreted by our adrenal glands when we're injured or under stress. These hormones are natural, cortisone-type healing and calming agents. Other steroids are secreted internally to control the body's sexual functions.

The steroids taken – unofficially – by some sports people are called anabolic steroids and can cause a temporary increase in the mass and tone of the muscles of the body, as well as the speed with which the muscles work. These should not be confused with topical steroids used to treat skin conditions. Having said that, the latter shouldn't be used on large areas of the body for a long time – say, daily for many weeks. Overuse of topical steroids, particularly the stronger ones and those applied to the face, may make the skin so thin that it can easily be damaged or will allow the active ingredient to pass through the skin and affect other parts of the body. Those most likely to be affected are infants and children, pregnant women, the elderly and people with kidney problems.

Topical steroids are particularly useful treatments for dry skin conditions such as eczema, dermatitis and psoriasis. They reduce redness and itchiness and help dampen down any inflammation. These creams contain topical steroids such as hydrocortisone, betamethasone (Betnovate range), clobetasone butyrate (Eumovate range), beclomethasone dipropionate (Propaderm range), or clobetasol propionate (Dermovate range), for example. Sometimes infection can also be a problem in these skin conditions. When this is the case, a topical steroid cream with an anti-bacterial agent and/or an anti-fungal agent can be effective, for example a cream such as Dermovate-NN Ointment which contains clobetasol propionate (a topical steroid), neomycin (an anti-bacterial agent) and nystatin (an anti-candidal agent).

Epogam

Epogam contains a special variety of evening primrose oil, the major active constituent of which is gamolenic acid, also known as gamma-linolenic acid (GLA). In order to perform its functions, linoleic acid, an essential nutrient, must be converted to GLA within the body. Research carried out by Scotia Pharmaceuticals showed that eczema sufferers fail to convert linoleic acid to GLA properly and do not make enough GLA for normal skin structure and function. Adding GLA to the diet can help correct this biochemical abnormality.

It's worth remembering that once the eczema improves the Epogam dosage may be reduced to a lower maintenance dose, but if treatment stops the patient's eczema may recur. According to the National Eczema Society, Epogam can take eight to twelve weeks before becoming effective. The main benefit appears to be a reduction both in the itchiness and in the need for steroids and antibiotics. So far no major adverse effects have been reported although nausea, indigestion and headaches have occasionally occurred.

Ultraviolet light

Severe cases of eczema may be treated with an ultraviolet light treatment similar to natural sunlight (a mixture of ultraviolet light A (UVA) and ultraviolet light B (UVB)), or with PUVA treatment – medicines known as psoralens given before treatment with UVA (see page 49).

Antihistamines

Sometimes your doctor may prescribe antihistamine tablets when itching really does become unbearable or uncontrollable. Antihistamines generally block the effects of histamine, which is released by the tissues when they are inflamed by an allergy or inflammation, adding to, if not actually causing, many of the unpleasant symptoms, particularly the itching.

The main side-effect of the older antihistamines – like chlorpheniramine – is sedation. When a medicine causes drowsiness you shouldn't drive, operate machinery or work at heights, and you should avoid alcoholic drink. Alcohol or other medicines may also alter the way the antihistamine works.

Some sufferers and their doctors also prefer the use of medicated bandages which already have the prescribed medication soaked into them. The bandages have the added advantage of helping the sufferer resist scratching.

SELF-HELP TREATMENT

You can combat the dryness, itchiness and flakiness by preserving the moisture content of your skin. Avoid harsh or highly perfumed soaps or bath additives; instead, try using emollient (moisturising) soaps, creams and specially made bath oils. And when bathing use warm water instead of hot. These emollient products can be helpful when the skin becomes dry. Give your skin a good long soak so that it has a chance to absorb all the oils. (Moisturising bath oils can make the surface of the bath slippery, so do be careful when getting in and out.)

Examples of products you can buy over the counter include Cream E45, Diprobase, Diprobath, Emulsiderm Emollient, Evening Primrose Oil (products containing this may be soothing for dry skin conditions), Morhulin, Oilatum Emollient, Polytar Emollient, Probase 3 Cream, Sudocrem, Ultrabase and Unguentum Merck.

Hydrocortisone, as I explained earlier, provides anti-inflammatory action yet is the least potent topical cortico-steroid available. Using a mild hydrocortisone cream will ease discomfort by reducing inflammation, calming irritated skin.

For children at home, keep their skin away from direct contact with wool or other rough fabrics – choose soft, pure cotton instead. (Contact the National Eczema Society for a list of cotton-goods stockists.) Keep their fingernails short and use only gentle cleansing products suitable for infants.

Some parents have found that letting their child become involved in his own skin care regime helps him cope with the eczema. If he is old enough he can rub in cream on those areas of the body which are accessible, or he can pour his own emollients into the bath. Taking part in this way can help the child feel more in control of the problem.

If you suffer from contact dermatitis, protect your hands when using household cleansing fluids or chemicals, etc., and avoid contact with metals, dyes or even washing powders which may cause you problems. Using creams such as Savlon Barrier Cream or Codella can protect sensitive skin as they form a protective barrier against potential irritants.

If you're not sure of the cause of your condition, consult your doctor, who may choose to carry out some allergy tests. If you know what plays a contributory factor then, naturally, try to avoid it. Easier said than done, I know, in some cases. But if house dust – or more specifically the mite – irritates your skin, you can try to minimise the problem by frequently hoovering floors and furnishing, dusting with a damp cloth, having the curtains and blankets cleaned regularly, covering mattresses with a plastic cover and using pillows and duvets made from artificial fibres rather than feathers. Polished boards or 'lino' are less of a mite trap than carpets. Mites thrive in warmth, so keep the bedroom cool and well aired. Smaller objects, such as children's fluffy toys and even pillows, can be put into the deep freeze for twelve hours every so often as the mites cannot survive at that temperature.

Many sufferers have told me that they feel very guilty and very self-conscious about scratching. The itch is often so bad they can't avoid attacking it. When skin is scratched so much that it bleeds, it can become vulnerable to infection, which in the long run only exacerbates pain and discomfort. The trick is to minimise the damage so keep nails clean and short by filing daily (cutting leaves sharp edges).

Older children and adults may find that gently rub-

bing or pressing the itchy area is a satisfactory alternative to scratching. Applying moisturisers when there's
an urge to scratch will cool the skin – and reduce the
damage caused by the scratching. And no matter how
young or old someone is, distraction is always better
than shouting 'Stop it!'

I'm regularly asked if stress has any effect on eczema.
I believe it does – and I am *sure* that stress can't help any
skin problem and will only cause you to feel more uncomfortable about it. (See pages 40–3 for more about
dealing with stress.)

Eczema is a condition which can be aggravated by
heat. Some sufferers find that their skin becomes even
more irritated by sitting in a centrally heated room, for
instance. So if you find that this is true in your case, it's
wise to avoid any form of heat whenever you can – be it
sunlight or even a glass of alcohol (which makes us feel
hotter because it opens up the small blood vessels just
under the skin).

CASE STUDIES: SUE AND TOLA

While we are concentrating on how sufferers feel and
how they cope with their skin problem, we ought to
spare a thought also for those people who share their
lives with someone with a skin problem.

Sue, a thirty-five-year-old busy mum of two sons
aged seven and four, finds life very difficult at times.
Both her sons suffer from atopic eczema, as does her
schoolteacher husband.

My husband has suffered off and on all his life. More on
than off. At times he has been dreadful and has had two
hospital stays. He also suffers from asthma.

As a partner it's very difficult. My husband will sit and
scratch and I find that so irritating. I know he's uncomfortable and he's not always aware that he's scratching. He
scratches at night in bed and that's intensely irritating. I

don't think that I'm always as sympathetic as I could be.

Carrying out his job, which is demanding, is as much as my husband can do sometimes. When he goes to work he's so busy he has to forget about his skin problem, which I think is important. So when he gets home it takes over a bit. He becomes much more self-centred. He'd rather sit and read the paper than do anything else. He's also very irritable because he is uncomfortable. At the moment he is better than he's ever been and so our home life is much better too. But in our family there's always one person at a time who is not particularly good.

The children are also very uncomfortable all the time. The younger one doesn't sleep too well and it's only during the past six months that he has slept through the night. Sometimes I could be up six times in the night to see to him. He used to scratch so much that his cot sheets would be covered in blood. When he was a baby he would also scratch his face.

The older one gets very hot at night. He itches and he just can't get to sleep, then he gets over-tired and he scratches even more. We just don't get enough sleep because of eczema. When you're tired everyone's tolerance levels drops. Looking back I don't know how I've coped at times. I suppose you do because you have to but it's very difficult. When everyone is tired it puts a terrible strain on family life.

People have asked me why I don't go to sleep when the children are at school or playgroup. It's not as easy as that. You can't just switch off to order, and anyway there are things that you need or want to do during the day. Of course, I used to go to bed early but I found I would be lying there waiting for one of them to wake up.

For the children life can be difficult too. And Sue's husband has felt very guilty that their difficulties are his 'fault'.

My older son is at school. He's been quite lucky. There is another boy in his class with eczema and he hasn't been picked on, apart from one boy who says that he's got germs. He always points out my son's eczema. He does get upset by it, but he's good, he just gets on with things. And it's good at school because they keep cream in the classroom so that if their itching is bad they can go and put it on. My older son is an outgoing, confident child. Things could have been even worse if he hadn't been. I've made him go to school every day, even when he is uncomfortable, because keeping him at home would be a bad habit to get into. Of course, if he was *ill* I would keep him home.

Even though Sue's little boy copes well with school there are minor restrictions on his life which make him feel different.

Sometimes the children sit on a carpet but my son has to sit on a chair because the carpet would make him hot and then itchy. He doesn't like to be the odd one out but he gets on with it. There are so many little things about eczema that add up to make life difficult.

Many people do not realise that being the odd one out is a serious problem for children. Doctors keep telling you they'll grow out of it – but in the meantime you've got to deal with it. My husband is thirty-five and he still hasn't grown out of it. It's only when you've coped with it yourself that you realise how difficult it is. Or people will say that it's only a bit of an itch. It is. But it's an itch all over your body so people ought to stop and think how difficult it makes the rest of your life. I do find people just don't understand.

Sue and her family try to cope with eczema as best they can by trying all manner of different treatments.

All we can do is to keep trying different things. We are careful about detergents, gas fires – for some reason they irritate my husband's skin more than electric fires. We haven't found any one thing in particular which triggers it off.

We use emollients such as E45 or Diprobase. We've found that you can get into a bit of a rut by using the same creams all the time. Sometimes just a change of emollient can make a big difference. At other times you know you ought to be trying different things but you just can't be bothered.

We've tried special diets. I don't think the family is

irritated by dairy products. Cutting out additives and food colourings, etc., seemed to help for a little while – although I would never have given the children cheap, horrible orange squash or fizzy sweets anyway. And they don't have cola drinks very often. Yet controlling their diet can be difficult when they go out to tea.

We've tried a medical herbalist and that was useless. Homoeopathic medicines which we have had prescribed on the NHS have helped my younger son. It's made a difference to his life and his skin is better, which means he can cope better. He's not scratching so much at night so he's not waking up as much.

Other self-help measures include wearing cotton clothing. I also keep their fingernails short. Talking of self-help measures, I do get annoyed when the first thing a doctor asks you is whether you have changed your detergent. They insult your intelligence. They trot out these questions without any thought that you might have read things about eczema or that you might be a member of the Eczema Society.

I have found that I have to be so strict with the children. I have to insist that they have a bath every night. They have to have their cream on. It's all an additional hassle. We have so much extra laundry because of eczema. Sometimes I have to change their bedding twice a week. They go through more clothes than other children because of the creams. I'm always washing my hands after putting on creams. We've just had water meters introduced in our area and I dread to think what our water bill is going to be.

When we go on holiday we have to take our own sheets. The family can only tolerate cotton ones. You have to think of so many little things – like not allowing the children to have their faces painted at a funfair or fête. Or when we went abroad recently and we had to take an airline bag full of medicines, moisturising creams, bath emollients, plus stronger creams just in case they were needed. We even have to be really careful about the suncreams we use!

Like Sue, twenty-seven-year-old Tola believes that coping with eczema is a matter of skin-care maintenance and working out what combination of treatments and measures helps you. She's had atopic eczema for the past nine years and says she never goes anywhere without Piriton antihistamine tablets and a tube of emollient cream.

Antihistamines don't really stop the itching but they make you drowsy and that helps you get some sleep.

I have to be so careful with my skin. It's quite dry anyway. I have to use moisturiser at least twice a day, sometimes more. I once spent three weeks in hospital. There I was given a mixture of liquid paraffin and white soft paraffin because my skin was so dry and it needed something very greasy. I've also used steroid ointments.

Using such greasy emollients has not been without its problems, though. Apart from extra washing, with clothes still coming out of the washing machine stained with grease, Tola has had plumbing problems.

We have had blocked drains three or four times a year from all the grease that gets washed down them. Now I make sure I pour hot water down the plug hole after having a bath.

But I have found that treatments never cure the condition. They just make it more bearable. I believe dealing with eczema is a question of maintenance. I always make sure I moisturise my skin. Even at work I have to go the loo to undress completely and moisturise my skin once a day. Sometimes I have to do it twice depending on how bad the eczema is.

I've tried a variety of ways of controlling my eczema, as the combination of emollients and steroid creams didn't seem to be improving things. Evening Primrose Oil made a tremendous difference at first. The itching stopped and my skin became smoother. Cutting out dairy products has helped a little. The effects weren't dramatic but enough to make me continue avoiding these foods. My skin became slightly smoother. Now I don't eat butter, yoghurt, milk, chocolate, cheese, anything with cream or milk or butter in, such as cakes. There are so many things which include dairy products in their ingredients.

I think eczema is a multifactoral thing. You have to combine the treatments that seem to work for you.

I couldn't put it better than that! Controlling the worst of the symptoms of eczema requires a combination of medical and nursing advice with a heavy sprinkling of what the sufferer finds works best for them.

3: PSORIASIS

Psoriasis is a common and painful skin condition affecting more than a million people in the United Kingdom and the Republic of Ireland. According to the Psoriasis Association, one in fifty people in the UK suffer from it. It can vary in severity from simply being a mild nuisance to being so bad that the sufferer has to be admitted to hospital (though I have to say this is rare).

Normally, the top layer of our skin has a self-regulating mechanism which replaces worn-out cells with just the right number of new ones. With psoriasis this replacement process gets out of control. Old cells are shed too rapidly and too many new ones are produced as the skin cells grow much faster than usual. In normal skin, the skin cells divide and shed every twenty-five to twenty-eight days. In cases of psoriasis this happens in just three to four days.

The precise cause of this isn't clear. There's evidence to suggest that it could be partly genetic, partly environmental. What is known is that a psoriasis attack can be triggered by stress (in someone who is susceptible to it), some drugs (beta-blockers prescribed for high blood pressure, for example) and even an infection with a virus, such as German measles, or some kind of injury to the skin, such as sunburn.

The most common form, plaque psoriasis, usually develops as scattered, raised, oval-shaped red patches with thick, silvery white scales. It mostly occurs on the knees, elbows and scalp. On the scalp it's noticeable as a thick white encrustation around the hairline and ears. The condition can become very painful on any part of the body liable to chafing.

As I've said, psoriasis seems to be linked to heredity – although there is no clear-cut pattern. Some experts believe that certain genes could be involved and that a person is more likely to inherit the *susceptibility* to psoriasis rather than the problem itself. According to the Psoriasis Association, if one parent has psoriasis, the chances of a child developing the condition are about one in ten. When both parents have the problem the child has a 50 per cent chance of developing it too.

Psoriasis affects men and women equally and can appear at any age, though it most usually develops between the ages of fourteen and forty-five, very often during adolescence, pregnancy and the menopause. As important hormonal changes are occurring at these times, it's likely that these play a part in the cause. The condition normally improves in the summer and gets worse again in the winter, due to the extra sunlight received by the body – one of the few occasions when sunbathing has a positive effect on the skin!

It can be a difficult condition to treat and, unfortunately, there's no long-term cure. Outbreaks tend to come and go – frequency and extent vary between individuals and cannot be predicted accurately. Although psoriasis is not usually harmful to general health and is not catching, the appearance of the skin can cause the sufferer great embarrassment and discomfort, particularly when large areas are affected.

A question I am often asked is whether psoriasis can disappear for ever. Patches will sometimes clear up for years but can then re-appear for no apparent reason. Unfortunately, it really is difficult to predict whether your psoriasis will go for good because it affects people so differently.

Psoriasis gives rise to many other questions, frequently: 'Is it true that a psoriasis sufferer can develop arthritis?' The answer is, yes. Psoriatic arthritis affects about 6 per cent of psoriasis sufferers. There's no link, however, between the location of the skin lesions and the location of the arthritic joints. In other words, the arthritis doesn't necessarily develop where the psoriasis is in evidence. This arthritis is a crippling condition which restricts movement, most commonly in the hands, elbows and back, as well as causing inflammation, pain and tenderness in any joint. Joints near the fingertips can often be affected, with the fingernails taking on a pitted look. It is a similar condition to rheumatoid arthritis although generally milder: other symptoms include morning stiffness and fatigue. Again, the cause is not known and sometimes it will disappear for no apparent reason, while in other cases it will linger on. There is just no way of telling, unfortunately.

Many of you will, I'm sure, recall the most extreme form of this skin condition in the popular television drama *The Singing Detective*. The leading character had exfoliative dermatitis, which can also be a serious complication of other skin conditions when they break out worse than usual. The leading character also had psoriatic arthritis and was bedridden.

Another question I am often asked is whether there is more than one type of psoriasis. Again, the answer is yes. As I've already mentioned, the most common form is plaque psoriasis, but there are other types:

• *Discoid psoriasis*, a common form, which causes patches of the characteristic white scales on a red background.

• *Guttate psoriasis*, where small (5–10 mm) scaly patches of skin appear all over the body, often after a bacterial throat infection or some other kind of infection.

• *Flexural psoriasis*, which appears in areas where there is a lot of skin contact, such as the armpits or buttocks.

• *Generalised pustular psoriasis*, which consists, as the name suggests, of small germ-free pustules (like small sterile boils) mainly affecting the hands and feet. This is a rare condition.

Another frequent question is why are there changes in a sufferer's fingernails and toenails? Most sufferers find that their nails are affected to some degree – they may grow extra fast and become thick and flaky, or become discoloured, or even pitted (making the surface of the nail look like the surface of a thimble). Also, the nail plate may become separated, though nails are rarely lost completely. This is because in psoriasis, the affected areas of skin show an abnormality in the way they mature. So the keratinisation process – the formation of the outer, hard, waterproof layer of the skin (which is the final part to mature) is disturbed. Why this should be so is not entirely understood.

Nails are an appendage of the skin – that is to say, they are produced in a similar way to the cells in the top layers of the skin, but have been modified to produce the more concentrated keratin which we know as the nail plate. This makes it easier to understand why any process which affects the skin as a whole, like psoriasis, can also affect the nails. Occasionally, changes to the nails may be seen where there are no other symptoms on the rest of the body.

People are often confused about the differences between psoriasis and eczema. And I am often asked, 'If a parent has psoriasis and her daughter develops eczema, does it follow that the two conditions are linked?' Well, psoriasis and eczema aren't specifically related, although both can run separately in the family. As I've explained previously, psoriasis is a condition in which the top layers of the skin are overproduced. This is usually seen as silvery flakes of surplus cells on top of a red, inflamed base of skin. Eczema is the name used to describe a *condition* of the skin – an eczematous reaction – rather than a specific disease.

TREATMENT

Although there is, as yet, no magical cure for psoriasis, the various treatments now available – which all aim to slow down the unusually rapid skin replacement and clear up the individual patches – can be very successful in improving a person's quality of life. *How* successful depends partly on an optimistic approach to treatment, partly on continuing supervision and encouragement in its use and partly on the sufferer's confidence in the doctor concerned. As is the case with many medical conditions, what suits one patient may not necessarily suit another.

On a day-to-day basis, emollient baths and creams (E45, for example) rubbed into the scaly patches can help to soothe the itching and flaking. Tar, or coal tar, can also be useful – in fact, coal tar ointments, baths and shampoos were once the only treatment available. Psoriderm Bath Emulsion is one you can buy from your local pharmacy. Alphosyl is another brand of lotion or cream containing coal tar, as well as allantoin for the treatment of psoriasis of the scalp.

Psoriasis is likely to respond to topical steroids (see page 22), but, unfortunately, once treatment is discontinued the psoriasis can return and, in some cases, worse than it was before, so this treatment will often be held in reserve.

Dithranol, a synthetic chemical, is administered in hospital and is an effective topical treatment for plaque psoriasis. Some sufferers describe this treatment as being bandaged up like a mummy. Newer creams and ointments containing dithranol have now become available (Psoradrate, Dithrocream, Dithrolan, Anthranol) so that treatment can be carried out at home (called short contact therapy). Sufferers tell me that these new treatments are an improvement on what went before but they still stain the skin, and bedding and clothing. For this reason treated areas are usually covered by tubular gauze in an effort to keep the drug off clothing. It is also an irritant and if not used carefully will actually burn the skin. The staining on the skin is only superficial, and will soon return to normal when the treatment is stopped.

A new treatment for psoriasis is Dovonex, an ointment which is usually applied twice a day to the affected areas (though not on your face). This ointment contains calcipotriol which helps to bring the excessive production of skin cells back to the normal level. The ointment shouldn't be used if you are allergic to any of the ingredients or if you know you've had problems with your calcium levels – since one of its known side-effects is to increase the body's concentration of calcium. And if your psoriasis gets worse, you should stop using the ointment and see your doctor immediately. You should not use it for more than six weeks at a time and it must not be applied to the face or scalp. Nor is it suitable for children.

Many members of the Psoriasis Association looked forward to the arrival of this new treatment but, unfortunately, it doesn't work for everybody. Some users complain that the treatment causes intense itching, others are not happy with the way the ointment 'burns off' the top layers of their skin. Some users find that it only gives them a temporary reprieve from psoriasis – although for many a temporary relief is still worth it.

But as Ray, a sixty-eight-year-old office worker explains, Dovonex does have advantages over other treatments because it does not smell and it doesn't stain clothing or skin.

I've had psoriasis for almost forty years and I've had every treatment going, from tar baths to dithranol, and I've had every ointment you can think of. I've had PUVA treatment which helped – everything seems to help but as soon as you stop the treatment the psoriasis returns anyway. I thought that when I retired the psoriasis might die down, particularly as it's said to be linked to stress. My consultant warned me not to bank too much on that and he was right. It hasn't happened that way and my treatment continues. I have to say that Dovonex is better than most treatments because it's not messy, it doesn't smell – it looks like petroleum jelly – and it's easy to apply. It keeps my psoriasis under control as long as I carry on using it.

PUVA therapy, which is a treatment sometimes offered to vitiligo sufferers, may help slow down the psoriatic process and can be quite effective (see page 49).

For severe, extensive psoriasis which is resistant to other forms of therapy, a medicine such as Neotigason (acitretin) may be prescribed. This is a vitamin A derivative. It could harm an unborn child, so women who may become pregnant shouldn't take this medicine, and contraception should be used for at least a month before treatment, all through treatment and for at least two years afterwards.

Most frequent side-effects of Tigason are dryness of the mouth and lips, itching, hair thinning and hair loss (alopecia) – which is reversible when treatment is stopped. Sometimes the levels of blood fat rise as a result of the drug, and will need to be monitored by regular blood tests.

Methotrexate is another powerful drug used to treat only the very severest psoriasis. It works by blocking cell division. However, this type of treatment can cause liver damage.

Over the counter you can by all sorts of moisturising creams and emollients. Other treatments that are useful are Danapharm Evening Primrose Oil products available in health shops, which can be soothing and help prevent further water loss, and you may find Dead Sea Bath Salts beneficial. See also the products listed under eczema (pages 25–6).

You can buy homoeopathic remedies from health shops and some pharmacies. Those said to be useful in psoriasis are *Arsen Alb*, *Graphites* and *Sulphur*.

PSORIASIS AND STRESS

Many people suffering with psoriasis find that their skin problem becomes worse if they're worried or under pressure. Often this can be a vicious circle, for when their psoriasis deteriorates it can make them worry even more.

However some experts believe that while there does seem to be a link between stress and psoriasis relapses, getting rid of stress might not improve the condition.

Measuring stress can be difficult. Stress to one person may not be stress to another, and some of us are naturally more sensitive to it than others. Yet when there is too much stress in our lives we can be creating all manner of problems for ourselves. (And that includes those of us who don't suffer from psoriasis.) Recognising (a) that we are stressed and (b) why we are stressed, and then acting to solve the problem isn't easy. However, stress isn't always a bad thing. Positive stress, or pressure, is needed for us to work well and to drive us to make the most out of life. That rush of adrenaline stimulates and motivates.

Your personality and the way you're made can decide how much stress you can take – I'm sure many readers will have heard of the 'fight or flight' response of caveman. Our bodies have an automatic response to fear or pleasure, releasing the hormones adrenaline and noradrenaline. These cause the heart rate to increase as well as providing instant energy by releasing sugars and fats into the blood. Once we would either stay and fight the man or animal causing us stress, or alternatively we would run away. Such reactions aren't easy these days!

So, because we can't 'flee' or 'fight', the body's adrenaline is bottled up instead, and this is when stress becomes a bad thing.

You may not realise when you are under stress though. Symptoms can include tense muscles, headaches or palpitations, your breathing can suddenly get faster and you may find yourself taking many short breaths. You may get sweaty palms, feel restless, tense or exhausted and your sleeping patterns can change (whereas once you slept well, your night could become interrupted, or you find that you keep waking early). You may also find yourself constantly thinking of things that have happened in the past, times when you have been hurt or when hurtful things have been said to you. Another symptom is hypochondria, where you are troubled by a fear of being seriously ill. These are just a few of the many examples of stress symptoms.

The Health Education Authority suggests some simple ways to help cope with stress. One of these suggestions is to organise your time by making a list of what is most urgent and what is least urgent. Do things in that order and don't take on more work than you can handle. It's also important to make time for relaxing.

You can learn a simple relaxation technique such as the one I use: sit or lie down somewhere comfortable when you know that for about half an hour you're unlikely to be disturbed. Let your body sink right down into what's supporting it. Then tense and relax each part of the body in turn – paying attention to any muscles that feel tense. By the time you have worked through all your muscles you'll feel as if you're a rag doll with no bones or muscles at all. Then go through all your relaxed muscles, thinking about how each one feels, so that you can learn to recognise when your muscles are becoming tensed during a stressful time.

Another good way of reducing the stress is to look at your lifestyle as if you were a fly on the wall. And remember, taking control of your life means dealing with one problem at a time. It's often easier for someone on the outside to work out what's causing you stress, which is why it's worth listening to another opinion – if you value that person's opinion, of course.

Discussing something that might be worrying you or

that has worried you in the past is another way of coping with stress. Talking through emotional problems can be the first step towards dealing with them. Naturally, you may prefer to talk to a trained therapist or counsellor but sometimes a chat with someone you respect can be just as helpful. It may be an old saying, but I think there's still value in it – a problem shared is so often a problem halved.

It's so important for you to realise that you don't have to cope on your own. If you keep whatever's troubling you to yourself, the shame and guilt involved in keeping it hidden can reinforce the problem. By talking things through with someone you're asking them to *listen* to you not solve your problems. I firmly believe that facing up to problems and talking about them is a sign of strength not weakness.

There are also other ways you can learn to relax and cope with stress. Yoga, for instance, may be worth a try. This has been practised in India for centuries as a means of maintaining health through the release of physical and mental tension. It can improve posture by training you to breathe properly and become flexible and supple, at the same time heightening your awareness of each part of your body as you stretch as far as you can without risking injury.

Yoga seems to be undergoing a resurgence of interest recently and it is believed to be an excellent means of managing stress because it is so calming. As you think about what's happening to your physical self, you have less tension and wipe from your mind jumbled thoughts and emotions. Nevertheless, don't rush into things if you start a yoga class, take it slowly but surely.

Meditation is another relaxation technique and hypnotherapy may also be useful. Holidays, too, are a good way of relaxing, especially in the sun – which is itself extremely beneficial for the relief of psoriasis. By encouraging a calmer outlook a trip away may even help prevent further outbreaks. In fact, some sufferers fly out to the Dead Sea for the beneficial effects of the environment. The haze which hangs over that part of the world screens out harsh UVB rays while the remaining UVA sunshine is extremely good for the skin. For many people the most important aspect of this sort of communal treatment is the realisation that they are not the only ones with the condition. They need no longer feel any shame or embarrassment about slipping into a swimming costume because so many other people there suffer from the condition. I've been fortunate enough to visit the Dead Sea psoriasis 'spas' and I've seen the sufferers arrive close to despair. Within a day or so, though, they're smiling, and a day or so after that their attack has all but disappeared. Fantastic.

This is one of the few occasions when, as a doctor, I feel able to recommend the sun for the skin. With psoriasis, its advantages can heavily outweigh the disadvantages. Indeed, if a sufferer's doctor or specialist were to recommend a sun lamp, I would consider that another acceptable treatment. However, you should ask for advice on the amount of time spent under the lamp, and the lamp should be of good quality so that it gives out more of the softer UVA rays and less of the harsher, burning UVB rays.

Remember, if you find that stress affects your psoriasis, peace of mind is essential in beating the condition.

PSORIASIS AND DIET

Sufferers can also benefit from eating more fish, especially oily types like mackerel and herring. It's been suggested that one of the unsaturated fats in fish oils, EPA, is able to replace another unsaturated fat called arachidonic acid. It is thought that the body's use of this last acid is upset in someone who suffers from psoriasis.

But despite all these possible remedies, active outbreaks should always be seen by a doctor. If the psoriasis is widespread or persistent, specialised hospital treatment will be recommended.

SUPPORT GROUPS

Many sufferers believe that talking to other sufferers helps them enormously. One person I know had endured psoriasis for ten years without ever meeting another sufferer. By chance a newspaper headline changed her life. It read: 'The P is silent and so are the sufferers.' The article led her to a meeting of psoriasis sufferers in her area.

For many people, the peace of mind that comes from knowing they are not alone is essential to beating the condition. Acceptance of the problem and learning how to live with it is also important.

CASE STUDY: SHEILA

Sheila, a fifty-four-year-old stock controller for a shoe company, has had psoriasis for forty years. She has learned to live with it and as she has got older has become less embarrassed by it. Nevertheless there have been times when she would not have wished psoriasis on her worst enemy and times when she has wanted to shrivel up with embarrassment because of it.

Psoriasis first appeared as a teenager but in a different form to what I have now. I had no idea it was psoriasis. Little tiny white blisters appeared on the palms of my hands and on the soles of my feet. They burst and left a scaly appearance to the skin.

Nobody ever told me I'd had psoriasis all those years ago. I lost my parents in my teens – my father when I was fourteen and my mother when I was fifteen. I had a nervous breakdown and then the psoriasis developed. My doctor told me it was all part of that. In my twenties it cleared up but then I developed discoid psoriasis. I was really upset when this new skin problem developed and the doctor told me, for the first time, that I had psoriasis and that I would just have to live with it. I was so angry I told him he ought to experience it and try to live with it. He sent me to a dermatologist after that. That's when I joined in group discussions about the disease and I found that helped enormously.

In a way my doctor was right, you do just have to live with it. But you don't always want to accept that fact. I think trying to accept it makes it easier to cope with. For me psoriasis was very difficult to live with initially. It seems that everyone around you has perfect skin. I think summertime is difficult for a woman with a skin problem, particularly if you have psoriasis on the areas that are revealed by summer dresses, such as legs, arms, hands.

I wouldn't ever wear a swimming costume. Now I don't care who says what, but when you're younger you just want to be the same as everyone else. You want to be part of the group and not appear any different. These days I can accept that I am who I am. In my generation you conformed. I remember going on a work outing many years ago. I stood in our hotel bedroom and told my husband that I couldn't possibly go downstairs in a swimming costume. Everybody knew I had psoriasis but nobody had seen me without clothes. It sounds silly but it took all the courage I had to go down. And nobody said anything.

Other people have not shown as much understanding or tact. She recalls one situation which hurt her deeply.

I had used my local newsagent's for many years. The first type of psoriasis I had was on the palms of my hands so you could hide it from people. But now I have it on the tops of my hands. When it's bad my mother-in-law has described it as looking like raw meat. It was bad on this particular day when I went into the newsagent's. Normally I wore gloves when it was bad but on this day I hadn't. When I handed over the money to the assistant I saw her back away because of my hands. I could have died on the spot.

It was at times like this that I felt that if my hands could have been chopped off I would have been OK. I know that

that's a wicked thing to think, because you would be completely lost without your hands, but I couldn't help it. To me that shows how desperate you can become when you have a skin problem. I even carry a card which says that psoriasis is not contagious. Most people also seem to associate skin disorders with a person being dirty, and that's one of the worst things to deal with.

I've tried all sorts of treatment – I've been wrapped in plastic and covered in ointment. My skin smelt like putrefying flesh – the most revolting smell I have ever experienced. It was a perfect breeding ground for any infection. The treatment helped cure the psoriasis but I ended up with nasty infections. Since then I have mainly used steroid ointments and creams.

Sheila finds that her psoriasis does wax and wane.

At the moment my psoriasis doesn't look too bad, yet it's driving me wild. The itching is unbelievable. I sometimes wonder whether it's better to have huge patches of psoriasis than this itching.

I know there's no cure and there have been times when I've just had enough. I ignore it and don't even put on any creams or ointments. Then I'll really go to town and religiously put on my ointments. Sometimes they do help. I'll use Betnovate 1:4, then Alphosyl. I have had dithranol treatment as an out-patient but it was so time-consuming. I had to go to the hospital every morning for an hour, before going to the office, or in the evening after coming home from work. So that was an hour out of every day just for having ointment applied and then being bandaged. The treatment stains clothes and bed sheets so I always use old bedlinen. And now I make sure I always have a sheet under my duvet as an additional protection, to save messing up the duvet cover all the time. The dithranol did help but I found that once I stopped the psoriasis came back worse than ever.

You try hard not to let psoriasis rule your life but that's difficult when the treatment itself impinges so much on your life. If you're not married it must be hard. I'm fortunate in that it hasn't changed my life but I do know people who haven't got married just because of their psoriasis. I know some of these people would have made good partners and good mothers. I think it affects people's self-esteem and that's upsetting. Psoriasis alters your life. Some people find acceptance hard, and there's no doubt about it, there is a shame attached to a skin problem. You feel ashamed because it's so easy for strangers to see that you have a problem.

For Sheila one of the worst things about psoriasis is that it's linked to heredity, and not only her son but now also her young grandson has the condition.

I tell him that it's nothing like Nanny's and that his is going to get better. I don't want him to know at the age of seven that he's probably going to have something like that for the rest of his life. For me that's the most upsetting thing about this skin problem – seeing my grandson develop it.

The doctor told my grandson that he was special to have psoriasis. Yet if we are honest it's horrible and we don't like it. If your skin is normal you don't even think about it, apart from when you put on sun lotion. Whereas when you have a skin complaint you are constantly aware of the problem. Nobody thinks about the natural covering of their body unless there is something the matter with it.

4: VITILIGO

Yet another common skin problem is vitiligo. Figures published by the Vitiligo Society estimate that more than half a million people in the UK and around 50 million people worldwide are affected.

Vitiligo causes patches of skin to turn white as pigment cells 'disappear'. These uneven patches can be very noticeable, particularly in those with darker skin. For black and Asian people in particular, the emotional trauma of the condition can be enormous. The fact that nobody knows what triggers it only adds to the distress. On top of this, the complaint can cause much physical discomfort as the skin is no longer properly protected against the sun's harmful rays.

Vitiligo can cause great trauma when it develops in childhood, as it so often does. And as we all know, children can be very cruel, not realising the distress their teasing and tormenting can cause. So not only does a child have to cope with the unusual appearance of their skin, they have to cope with the extra strain of being made fun of. That's why it's important for a child to understand what is happening to his or her skin and why he or she looks different.

As I said, the condition is caused by the pigment cells in the skin – those normally responsible for making skin darker – simply stopping working. Though nobody seems to know for sure, there are a number of theories as to why this happens. Some people think that a chemical factor in the skin inhibits the production of the pigment cells. Others suggest that the cells are destroyed by a build-up of toxic substances within them. But the most popular theory is that vitiligo is an auto-immune disease – that is, the body's defences turn on the pigment cells as they would an invading germ. (Other theories include trigger factors such as stress, injury and hormonal changes.)

As with so many conditions that have an unknown cause, the only conclusion one can reach is that some people – and sometimes families – are more susceptible than others.

TREATMENT

There is no definite cure for vitiligo, but there are various treatments. The most common – steroid creams and PUVA (see below) – are available on the NHS. These may help some sufferers, but be warned that sadly they don't work for everyone. You really need to consult a dermatologist on the type of treatment that may be best suited to you.

Steroid creams similar to those used by eczema sufferers (such as Efcortelan, Synalar, Betnovate to name just a few) can enhance repigmentation when applied to the affected areas. But steroids can only be used for short periods at a time as they may produce side-effects, such as a thinning of the skin. No one really knows why they work – the obvious explanation is that there may be inflammation present, which the steroids, as powerful anti-inflammatory medicines, dampen down and so allow re-pigmentation to occur. However, I remain sceptical of this idea since the skin of most sufferers rarely shows any signs of inflammation.

PUVA is a treatment requiring the long-term use of ultraviolet A light in conjunction with Psoralen, a natural substance found in certain plant seeds. The medicine can be given by mouth or applied directly on to the skin. This treatment increases the beneficial effects of ultra-violet light but no one really knows how it works to restore pigmentation. It is known to react with DNA – the gene chemical at the centre of the cells in our body – but it is also suggested that pigment from deeper down in the skin is encouraged to migrate upwards into those parts of the skin where it can be seen. This treatment is not necessarily suitable for all vitiligo sufferers, and the results can never be guaranteed.

PUVA treatment is not without its side-effects, either. These can include the risk of the skin burning when exposed to sun, even through windows or glass. There may also be a small risk of skin cancer, malignant melanoma, particularly in those with light-coloured skin. All potential patients are therefore asked to sign a consent form before treatment begins. However, the risk is really no greater than someone with normal skin spending two weeks in a very hot climate in the full glare of the sun – something many of us do without giving a second thought to the danger. If treatment is given orally, nausea, itching, erythema (redness) or a skin reaction similar to a burn can result.

For the minority who do undergo PUVA, it is most important to approach it with a sensible attitude. Try not to get impatient – the treatment must be allowed to run its full course to have its proper effect. Pace yourself, closely observing your body's reactions. And, as with any medical treatment, talk to the consultant so you understand what it entails.

At the moment, research is being carried out into the treatment of small patches of vitiligo by transplanting either sections of normal skin or melanocytes (pigment cells) which have been grown in a test tube. Both of these treatments may hold hope for the future but they are still at the experimental stage, and they can only be used to treat very small areas.

Other research, carried out in Italy, concerns the taking of certain nutrients – called anti-oxidant therapy. Medical research can now support what some nutritional experts have been saying for years – that certain food components play a vital role in protecting us from disease. The nutrients concerned are trace minerals, such as selenium, and certain vitamins, particularly A, C and E.

Selenium is found in bread and cereals, mushrooms, garlic and Brazil nuts; vitamin A in carrots; vitamin E in green, leafy vegetables, as is vitamin C which is also found in citrus fruits. Past research has suggested that a regular supply of these nutrients could protect against heart disease and recent research has shown that patients taking pills containing selenium and vitamins A and E over a five-year period lived longer and had fewer episodes of cancer than those not taking the pills.

I've no doubt that we shall hear more about natural cures in the future so I was not surprised to learn of anti-oxidant therapy for the treatment of active vitiligo. Eating a diet rich in the anti-oxidants mentioned above will be beneficial, but it is also thought necessary to take them as regular dietary supplements. When they are taken in this way they are more likely to be referred to as anti-oxidant therapy, implying that they will be curative.

The therapy is based on a theory that certain stress hormones of the adrenaline type may cause 'oxygen starvation' in the skin tissues which, as a result, over-produce harmful chemicals called oxy-radicals, among others. It is claimed that these harm the pigment cells and so cause vitiligo, without leading to other immediate or obvious harm to the body as a whole. Recent trials suggest that there may be justification for optimism and further reports are awaited.

But what can be done now? On the whole little to bring back the lost colour. The use of camouflage cosmetics under professional guidance is often the best answer. Using such camouflage creams can give a sufferer just that little bit of extra confidence. Cosmetics are usually water-resistant and likely to be most successful on the face as it is difficult to apply make-up to larger areas of the body. The Red Cross Beauty Care and Camouflage service can provide excellent advice and support on this – but you'll need a letter of referral from your GP. Some camouflage products are available on prescription. These are called Covermark (Cupharma),

Dermacolor (Charles H Fox), Keromask (Innoxa) and Veil (Thomas Blake and Co.).

While a small amount of sunshine is beneficial – it supplies vitamin D and helps to keep at bay the more harmful germs that live on the skin – there is no longer any doubt that continuous and prolonged exposure to the sun or the rays of a sunbed can be harmful, causing dryness, blemishes, and, as we get older, wrinkles and loss of elasticity (see page 85). Each time the skin is burnt, the damage accumulates and the risk of skin cancer developing in the future increases.

Over-exposure to the ultra-violet rays of the sun makes the skin red, hot and sore. Higher doses lead to inflammation and swelling; and even greater exposure leads to burning, blistering and peeling, as the epidermis disintegrates. Very bad sunburn damages our skin so much that it cannot carry out its normal functions, for example the heat absorbed from over-exposure to the sun can stop the body's temperature gauge from working properly, resulting in sunstroke, which has been known to kill.

Although it is perhaps of little comfort to extreme vitiligo sufferers, their lack of pigment cells does mean that they are less likely to develop skin cancers that are caused by pigment cells – malignant melanomas. Though this doesn't mean that the sun poses no threat to them – because of their reduced amount of pigment, which is one of the skin's main protective factors, sufferers of vitiligo do have to take special precautions when exposing themselves to the sun. Avoiding exposure to the hot sun, as well as using high-protection sun creams, is vital. Non-pigmented skin does develop some protection – the top rough layer of skin thickens – but, in itself, this is not enough.

At least vitiligo isn't always painful or debilitating, and sometimes does get better with the passage of time. Unfortunately, however, this happens all too infrequently.

CASE STUDIES: JACQUELINE AND MAXINE

Many sufferers agree that accepting that you have vitiligo is an important part of coping with the condition. Jacqueline, a nineteen-year-old degree student, has suffered from vitiligo since she was ten years old.

I had a tiny patch of white skin on my chest which appeared after I had a red rash called pityriasis rosea [see page 81]. It was only about two centimetres across. About a year later small patches appeared on both knees which were roughly symmetrical. We have family photograph albums and you can see how the vitiligo progressed with each family holiday.

I now have no pigment at all on my hands, my elbows are white, the inside of my arms on the joints, my face is white, my knees, feet and hips are affected and it all seems to be symmetrical.

We happened to see something on television about the Vitiligo Society, which we joined when I was twelve. It was good for me as I'd thought that I was the only person. I was tender at that age – I was just beginning to develop, my periods had just started and I felt very alone. It helped to see other people with the condition and to realise that it wasn't that bad after all.

I have been lucky, I haven't been teased by friends. I have had some problems with strangers, though. People would stare and children would sometimes seem surprised and tell me that my skin looked funny. I had a stupid comment a couple of years ago from an adult. He asked me what was wrong with my skin and told me that it looked as if I had Tipp-Ex all over it. I couldn't believe such a comment from someone who was supposed to be an adult. I was so embarrassed.

Jacqueline found the Vitiligo Society was helpful to her in many ways.

After joining the society I wore one of its T-shirts which says, 'Help find a cure for vitiligo'. This gave me more confidence, as if it were a badge and therefore I didn't have to explain to strangers what was wrong with my skin. These days I don't mind so much but it did bother me when I was younger. Although I still don't like people looking at my skin or talking about it too much. Now I tell myself that there are things that are far worse, especially other skin diseases, and that's how I cope.

I also make sure that I am very careful about going out in the sun. I love cycling and I have to be careful with my hands in particular. I have been careless a couple of times and have been burnt and had swollen eyelids. I make sure I always use high-protection factor sunscreens. I like the ones the Body Shop sell. I always make sure I put on the lotions before I go out in the sun. I suppose one advantage of having to be so careful in the sun means when I get older my skin won't have aged so much.

I think coming to terms with vitiligo makes you a better person. If people don't like you for what you are and just look at your skin rather than your personality then they're not worth knowing. Someone who likes you for what you are is a much nicer person. I was given that advice when I was about thirteen and it's a nice way of putting it.

Maxine Whitton, a fifty-three-year-old academic librarian who has taken early retirement and who is also chair of the Vitiligo Society, first developed the condition when she was ten after a little appeared on her knees and forehead. She believes the disease can cause immense distress to sufferers and that a lot more money for research is needed.

My vitiligo has had an erratic course. By my teens it had spread to my eyes, lips and neck and then it became a problem for me. I was brought up in Jamaica. I had PUVA topically which helped repigment some of my skin but I couldn't do it for long because of the risks involved. While I was at college in England it started to spread further.

Maxine was fortunate in that she was shown how to apply camouflage creams properly and for her this was an excellent way to cope with the problem.

I have always used camouflage creams. It's very difficult to interact socially if people are distracted by the blotches on your face. I was shown how to apply it properly by a Mayfair salon. I've always had it prescribed. It's brilliant. It's so successful because my skin texture has not been changed. I'm also fortunate in that there is a shade that exactly matches my skin. I have a darker one again for use in summer. It gives me a lot more confidence and I never go out without it.

Because my vitiligo did not spread very rapidly I could pretend I was all right and I could hide behind creams. When I got to about forty it began to spread all over my body. I panicked because I felt it was taking over and that it was out of control. I had to face the possibility that I was going to lose all the pigment in my skin. As a black person I could not bear that idea. I became very depressed.

In my thirties I didn't bother going to hospital. I used make-up and adapted my clothes. I would wear long sleeves in summer and got fed up of people asking me whether I was hot. Of course I was hot. I decided to buy clothes to cover up my body. I spent a lot of money on clothes, I suppose to boost my confidence and to compensate for having to wear sleeves all the time.

I think you have to come to terms with yourself as someone with vitiligo and with the fact that your appearance is changing all the time. It's a progressive disfigurement which is not the same as a birthmark. I feel people trivialise it by saying it's just your skin. But socially and psychologically it can be quite a problem. You can't tell a person who has a headache, well, aren't you lucky you don't have toothache!

I had counselling when I had family problems and the vitiligo was spreading. My self-esteem was down to the ground. I had nine months of counselling that helped to give me some self-confidence and focus on the fact that vitiligo is a small part of my entire self and to be positive about other parts of my life. There are people who still deny vitiligo is a problem for them. Denial is a stage you go through. Acceptance is quite hard. My vision of myself is as one colour. You grieve because you have lost something. It's the same with any skin disease. I think there are people who don't face up to it and say it doesn't bother them. But it doesn't bother them because they don't face up to it.

I'm sure something will be done one day. There is exciting research going on. The problem is we don't have the money in this country to fund the research we'd like. I feel dermatology is so far down the list for funding. Yet skin is the biggest organ in the body, which keeps the outside out and the inside in. It's really not given enough importance.

5: AN A–Z OF OTHER SKIN PROBLEMS

As well as the main skin problems we've discussed in this book, I am very often asked to explain other common, and not so common, skin conditions. So I thought it would be useful to include some examples here.

ANAL ITCHING

Itching around the anus (back passage) is a common problem and is known medically as pruritis ani. It is slightly more common in men and people often put up with it for years, trying various self-help remedies (which may do more harm than good) because they are too embarrassed to consult their doctor. In fact, doctors are well used to examining this area and do not think twice about it. If sufferers could only realise this and overcome their embarrassment, much unnecessary discomfort could be prevented. Also, pruritis ani can be a symptom of an underlying condition, such as diabetes or an infection, for which treatment is required, so if you have this kind of itching, it really is important to be examined by a doctor.

Often, however, the condition is brought about by the sufferer himself. For instance, research has shown that people who tend to worry about their bowels, and take laxatives to keep them regular, are particularly prone. The laxatives, especially liquid paraffin, may cause leakage, or several bowel movements a day. Excessive amounts of high-fibre foods can have the same effect. Frequent wiping or washing then becomes necessary and this can soon chafe the skin and set up a constant irritation. Some people become obsessed about disinfecting or deodorising the area, using quite strong solutions that can make matters worse. Laxity of the anal sphincter (the normally tight band of muscle at the exit) can also lead to leakage and consequent irritation. So too can frequent straining to pass a motion, or increased pressure within the rectum, due to piles, for example.

Other conditions that can lead to a rectal discharge and irritation include an anal fissure or fistula, Crohn's disease, genital warts and a polyp – a small, benign growth. A vaginal discharge due to an infection, such as trichomonas, can also affect the anal region and cause pruritus.

The anal area, being warm and moist, is prone to infections, such as the fungus which also causes vaginal thrush (see page 72). This infection is more likely to thrive in overweight people whose skin often becomes chafed, but an anti-fungal cream prescribed by the doctor usually clears this up quickly. Overweight people also tend to sweat more which adds to any irritation as the anal skin is richly supplied with itch spots that are aggravated by warmth. A cool bath or bidet will usually relieve the itching or at night, when it is often at its worst, bathing the area with a damp sponge can be very soothing.

Threadworms are another cause of itching, as is, though much more rarely, scabies (see page 82). And, of course, skin conditions, such as eczema and psoriasis, can cause irritation around the anus. Sometimes the condition will simply occur following a course of antibiotics. Some people are sensitive to soaps, deodorants and biological washing powders and these can lead to dermatitis and recurrent episodes of intense itching. It will be a question of trial and error to see which, if any, is affecting you.

It often helps to shave the area as this reduces

chafing, and cotton underpants are best. Calamine lotion can be soothing. After a bowel movement, bathe the area with lukewarm water, with no antiseptics added. Avoid scratching if at all possible and do not rub in creams or ointments too vigorously.

As you can see, there are many possible causes for this kind of itching so do consult your doctor for a definite diagnosis as the condition can be made worse if, say, the wrong type of cream is used. Most of the problems settle down with suitable treatment. You should inform your doctor if you have a known sensitivity to local anaesthetics because he may wish to prescribe a suppository treatment, many of which contain a mild anaesthetic. Topical corticosteroids may also be prescribed. Just occasionally symptoms persist and then referral to a specialist will usually be recommended.

BACTERIAL SKIN PROBLEMS

Boils

Boils, sometimes called furuncles, are usually due to a bacterial infection of the skin and are extremely painful. The boil usually starts in and around a hair follicle where skin cells are destroyed by bacteria. Pus then develops, building up such pressure that the boil can burst.

Folliculitis

This condition presents itself as a small collection of discrete red pimples, some of which may have a yellow 'head'. It can occur anywhere on the body where there are hair follicles – i.e. everywhere except the palms of the hands and the soles of the feet. It is the result of a slightly more virulent germ than usual getting into one of these hair roots, and then, once established, propagating and spreading to other follicles. It's likely that the germs are no more harmful than the usual germs on the skin, but have just become established and entrenched. They not only live in hair follicles but also breed in the warm and moist places in the body, just inside the nose and between the cheeks of the bottom, for example.

Impetigo

Impetigo is a highly contagious skin problem which mainly affects children. It can spread very quickly, which is why, if you suspect your child has it, you should see your GP as soon as you can. It can sometimes be an additional problem for a child who suffers from eczema as the already inflamed skin is an easier target for the germ which causes it – the Staphylococcus Aureas bacteria.

Paronychia

This is usually due to a bacterial infection occurring in the skin at the side of a nail – on the fingers or toes – which produces a throbbing type pain as pus gathers often under the nail itself. It is treated with antibiotics, and if an 'ingrowing' nail is cutting into the tissues, this will be corrected by trimming the nail, permanently, down the appropriate side. The sufferer will also be told to keep the nails trimmed straight across, as cutting around a nail can cause sharp edges at each corner which can rub into the skin and allow germs to enter more easily.

Whitlow (or felon)

This is often confused with a paronychia. A whitlow is an infection, again usually bacterial, which affects the pulp, or pad, at the fingertip (whereas a paronychia is an infection of the tissues at the side of the nail). Until treated, either with antibiotics or by a small incision to let out the pus, a whitlow can be very painful because pressure builds up when the pus cannot escape either through the fairly thick skin here or through the nail plate itself.

Treatment

For bacterial skin conditions such as boils, impetigo and folliculitis, your doctor may prescribe an antibiotic ointment. Or sometimes you'll need to take a course of antibiotic tablets, such as penicillin, flucloxacillin or cloxacillin.

Topical antibiotic medicines can sometimes sting, burn or cause itching sensations when they are applied. When such ointments are used on the face, extra care should be taken to avoid getting any in your eyes.

BIRTHMARKS

Birthmarks, as the name implies, are with us from the day we are born although they are not always visible from the start. They arise from naevoid cells, and, as a rule of thumb, the different types of mark are caused by these cells lying in different areas of the skin. For example, if naevoid cells lie in the pigmented layer of the skin – among those cells that make you go brown when you lie in the sun – then the birthmark will be a brown one.

Sometimes a birthmark will appear many years after birth. When it is shown to a doctor – as it often is because it can cause great anxiety – he or she will call it a naevus (another name for a birthmark). The mark may only show up when that part of the skin is exposed to the sun.

The brown birthmarks can be flat or raised, or knobbly with hairs growing out of them. They differ in appearance according to where the 'root' of the naevoid cells happens to be.

However there are many other forms of birthmark:

Pigmented naevus (or mole)

It's funny to think that only twenty to thirty years ago, having a brown birthmark on the cheek was considered attractive. Women would stain them darker and call them beauty spots, so they're not all bad!

Many of the small, barely visible brown marks on our body, better known as freckles, are really birthmarks. On average, we all have about thirty of them (though to get that average means some of us are 'covered' in freckles, while others have only one or two). When the brown ones are unsightly, bleaching creams from pharmacists or camouflage make-up can be effective.

Port-wine stain

I think this is probably the most distressing of all birthmarks. It is caused by a cluster of tiny arteries, veins or capillaries (the very smallest of the blood vessels) which may cover a large area and colour it a port wine shade, hence the name. The marks are mostly just flat discolourations although they may also rise above the surrounding skin.

At the moment the use of argon lasers continues to provide one of the best available permanent treatments. Lasers produce light in a concentrated form. (For the scientific minded, it produces a beam of one wavelength and in just one plane, whereas normal light is produced in all planes, that is to say through the whole 360 degrees.) Consequently, very high amounts of light energy can be focused on to one spot and used to cut through tissues. A wavelength that is best absorbed by the tissues to be targeted is chosen. It will destroy these marks specifically, but leave the surrounding tissues as complete as possible and, hopefully, with minimum scarring.

Spider naevus

These are small red star-shaped spots that look rather like a very small red spider. They are due to an enlargement of the small veins and appear in twos and threes on the face or hands of children. They may also arise in adults 'out of the blue'. They are numerous during pregnancy and with serious liver disease (they will usually disappear soon after delivery or if the liver condition improves).

Sometimes these marks can just disappear spontaneously, although electro-cautery to the centre of the blemish with a hair-fine instrument of the kind used to permanently remove hairs by electrolysis can be recommended.

Strawberry naevus

This is a red birthmark which usually appears on the head and neck at or soon after birth. In the majority of children, even the most remarkable of these marks can completely disappear by the time the child is four or so. When they do this naturally it is usually without trace, whereas trying to remove them earlier is far more likely to leave a scar.

Many birthmarks cause no problems at all. They're not particularly noticeable, they don't get in the way and they cause no symptoms. When they do cause symptoms – for instance, start to itch, bleed, change colour or increase in size – then it's always wise to consult your doctor.

BLOOD BLISTERS

Blood blisters may be flat in appearance and look just like a leak of blood immediately under the skin – which is exactly what they are. They rise above the surface when the pressure of the blood forces up the skin's top layers.

Treatment depends very much on the cause, which may be an allergy that interferes with the production of platelets or a blood disorder such as leukaemia which, by overproducing white cells, 'squeezes' these platelets out of the blood vessel. Platelets are important cells as they are used by the body to act like small 'sandbags' to plug up any tiny leaks in the blood vessels – caused, for example, as a reaction to medication or severe infection or through a fragility of the vessels themselves.

Blisters which suddenly appear in an otherwise young and fit person can be due to a condition known as purpura, which arises when the platelets are diminished in number. However, most often no apparent cause can be found for the blister and the condition clears up on its own.

Later in life, these red spots can occur spontaneously, and this condition is known as 'old age' purpura or senile purpura. In addition, smaller red spots which look like blood blisters can occur – these are called Campbell de Morgan's spots and are nothing at all to worry about.

CHILBLAINS

Chilblains – blistered, sore or pus-filled areas of skin – occur most frequently in the winter, and affect more women than men and more young women than old. Although they're due to a minor abnormality of the local blood circulation, the symptoms can be very distressing.

In extremely cold weather, burning, itching, pain and redness may arise on the fingers of those mildly susceptible to the condition. The fingers are the most vulnerable because they are more often exposed to the cold – gloves tend to be removed out of doors, which doesn't often happen with socks, tights and shoes!

At worst, the symptoms can arise in quite mild weather, and for such sufferers the whole period from November through to April can be a miserable time, especially if they don't take extra care to keep the hands and feet warm and to avoid extreme changes in temperature.

With chilblains it appears that the small blood vessels constrict in the tissues. This is a natural occurrence, as the body automatically supplies less blood to the skin surface in order to retain essential heat deep within the tissues. (For the body's functions to work, the kidneys, heart and especially the blood have to maintain a constant temperature of around 37°C/98.4°F.)

But with chilblain sufferers the small vessels remain shut down for longer than usual. When fingers or toes are exposed to warmth and become red, the ill-effects of the under-supplied skin tissue strike with a vengeance as the blood returns and normal sensations come back. This results in the pain which every sufferer knows only too well.

The best preventative measure for this condition is to find ways of keeping the worst-affected extremities warm. Battery-heated gloves and socks are able to supply a constant, minimum amount of heat which will help prevent those small blood vessels shutting down as the temperature drops.

When chilblains occur, especially in an extreme form, a doctor should be consulted. There are other causes of such symptoms, for example Raynaud's disease, which may require additional forms of treatment.

CYST, SEBACEOUS

These are rounded lumps on the skin which can become very painful. They are caused by a blockage to the entrance of the sebaceous gland, which produces the skin's sebum or oil and sits at the base of a hair root. The blockage is either due to a bunching up of the skin's cells around the entrance, or to a drying-out of the sebum as it reaches the surface air. The cysts can occur anywhere on the body where there are sebaceous glands – i.e. everywhere except the palms of the hands and the soles of the feet.

DANDRUFF

Dandruff is the most common cause of itching of the scalp, but is not a sign of general ill-health or poor hygiene. Normally, everyone's skin cells, including those on their scalp, are replenished about every twenty-eight days and the top layer sheds in minute, usually unnoticeable, pieces. In dandruff sufferers, this process may be speeded up and larger particles are shed, which can therefore easily be seen.

With milder forms of dandruff, sometimes known as scurf, the flakes of skin are dry and white and tend to clump together in the hair. Touching the hair – which most people do many times a day without realising – dislodges the fragments and they fall on to the shoulders, looking like a white powder. This type of dandruff can usually be controlled by washing the hair two or three times a week with a medicated, anti-dandruff shampoo. This often contains tar, sulphur or salicylic acid to soften and help loosen scale and scalp debris. Other anti-dandruff shampoos for more severe cases contain zinc pyrithione or selenium sulphide to reduce the development of dandruff by slowing down the growth of skin cells They also have mild anti-fungal properties. Antibacterial gels which contain benzalkonium chloride may also be useful.

There is, however, a more severe form of dandruff called seborrhoeic dermatitis of the scalp, which may not respond to these shampoos (see page 17). On a baby's scalp this is known as cradle cap (see page 67) and also often appears as a nappy rash for which your doctor can prescribe a cream.

Both seborrhoeic dermatitis and other forms of

dandruff were once thought to be caused by an over-production of sebum. Diet, hygiene, climate and stress were also believed to play a part. However, recent research has shown that it is caused by the sufferer's over-reaction to a minute, fungus-like organism called the Pityrosporum ovale. It is the *reaction* to the fungus, rather than the fungus itself, that causes the scalp's top layer of skin to flake off.

Fortunately, there is good news for sufferers whose symptoms are severe – a specific anti-fungal shampoo called Nizoral is available on prescription and is very effective.

Neither dandruff nor seborrhoeic dermatitis is catching, because, as I said, it is not the fungus itself that produces the symptoms – as it is with athlete's foot, for instance – but an over-reaction to it, which only occurs in susceptible people.

Cradle cap

Cradle cap is a harmless condition resembling dandruff that is extremely common in young babies. It usually appears during the first three months of a baby's life, but can also affect toddlers and young children. If your baby develops cradle cap, you may first of all notice a little scurf on his or her head, followed by the appearance of yellowish or brownish greasy-looking scales of thickened skin which stick to the scalp. These patches sometimes appear over the whole head, or sometimes just in small areas. Some specialists believe the crusts are due to excess production of sebum – grease from the sebaceous glands – in response to the mother's hormones.

You can ease cradle cap by rubbing your baby's head with baby oil or olive oil and leaving it on for twenty-four hours. Comb the hair gently, then wash the flakes of skin away. Alternatively, treat cradle cap with specially formulated shampoos available from your pharmacist.

DRY SKIN

While acne is common with the young, dry skin is common among the middle-aged and elderly. It often causes itchiness, tightness or red patches of chafed-looking skin (or all of these symptoms combined). These signs often cause anxiety as the sufferer sees them as symptoms of some awful disease rather than, quite simply, the skin drying out. So that's why I feel it's worth a mention here.

In cold countries – where the air in centrally-heated houses contains a fairly small amount of moisture – a large proportion of the patients visiting a skin specialist will have dry skin as the 'underlying' cause of their problem. An electric humidifier to replace the moisture in the air may help them considerably. What's more, it also stops any wooden furniture suffering!

The second line of defence is to protect the skin from other drying agents – such as the sun, the wind, very hot showers and swimming pools that have been over-chlorinated.

And now for the treatment . . . There's a whole range of moisturising preparations, some specially prepared to wash with, some to add to your bath water, and some to spread over your skin. The latter are mixed in such a way that they can be completely rubbed in, which prevents that greasy feeling and – worse still for the elderly in the bath – the slipperiness that can cause a fall. At the expensive end of the market, there are products that when held under the running tap will dispense the moisturising droplets evenly throughout the bath water to leave the skin feeling silky soft – a sign that it's been moisturised. Ask your pharmacist about these.

Preparations with little or no perfume in them are preferable, as some people's skin reacts to a whole range of substances – perfumes among them. Since aroma is not essential, why take the risk?

If your skin is feeling dry and itchy after your usual

bath or shower routine, it's time to take care of your skin. And it's not just the doctor talking now . . . I say this with some feeling, because a few years ago my own skin started to get dry. But if I hadn't told you, you'd never have known – because I take precautions and follow my own advice!

EPIDERMOLYSIS BULLOSA (EB)

This a rare and painful genetic skin disease which is caused, in simple terms, by the fibres holding the skin layers together not working properly. Estimates suggest that in this country some 2500 children suffer from EB. There are three types – simplex, dystrophic and junctional (the most severe of which can cause death within the first year of life).

The main symptoms are blisters which can appear as hugh water pouches arising from the skin, similar to those seen in someone who has been badly, though superficially, burned – as in the more severe forms of sunburn. These blisters are caused by fluid collecting in the gaps between skin layers. If any of these blisters are broken there is a much greater risk of an infection entering the body.

EXCESSIVE SWEATING

In my postbag I regularly receive letters from readers and listeners who are distressed by excessive sweating. They usually want to know whether there is some powerful, curative medical treatment which they could try.

I usually advise them to return to their pharmacist or GP, because I know that there are several good antiperspirants available – your GP may suggest one with aluminium chloride and aluminium hydroxide. Wearing clothes made out of natural materials, rather than synthetic, may also help. And it is a good idea to wash at least once a day with an anti-bacterial soap which will remove stale sweat and control bacterial growth.

Sweat is a secretion produced by microscopic sweat glands – we have about 2.5 million scattered under the skin's surface. They release moisture – sweat – through pores in the skin's surface to regulate body temperature. Sweat itself has no noticeable odour, but if it remains on the skin for more than a few hours it may begin to smell. This is caused by the bacteria which flourish in sweat, particularly that of the apocrine glands in the armpits, groin and nipples. (In fact, the dome of the armpit contains 80 per cent of our sweat glands.) The apocrine glands also produce perspiration and greater amounts of personal scent when we are sexually aroused.

It is true that some people sweat more than others, so if you've always perspired profusely there's unlikely to be anything wrong with you. However, perspiring that's not brought on by heat or exercise, which is much more profuse than you're used to, may be due to a medical condition. So always consult your doctor if this happens to you.

If you are still young, and feeling desperate about excessive perspiration, remember that the problem will lessen in time. As you feel more sure of yourself in public, and as those early emotional experiences diminish in their intensity, then the excessive sweating will as well.

FUNGAL SKIN PROBLEMS

Athlete's Foot

Athlete's foot (tinea pedis) is a fungal infection of the skin which thrives in warm, wet conditions. The skin between the toes becomes red, soggy, itchy, flaky and sometimes smelly. It's not very common in children but is a frequent problem for adolescents and sporty young men and women who use communal changing rooms. The condition will persist until it's treated and, as other people can be infected, prompt attention is required.

Treatment is fairly straightforward. If you suffer from athlete's foot – or as a precaution against it – you should ensure your feet are kept dry. 'Air' them as often as possible, wash them frequently, particularly during hot weather, change your socks or tights daily and avoid walking barefoot in public changing rooms. If you have to use a changing room or communal shower, wear sandals to avoid the risk of infection from the floor.

Anti-fungal creams, sprays or powders are usually very effective, applied on to and around the affected skin. Sprinkle the powder liberally on to the feet, particularly between the toes. It's helpful, too, to dust socks and the insides of shoes before wearing them. Unless the instructions on your medicine advise you differently, continue treatment for a week after all signs of infection have disappeared. If the condition doesn't clear up in a week or so, you may need a stronger anti-fungal agent than those available over the counter.

Ringworm

Despite its name, ringworm is a fungal skin infection, and has nothing to do with worms. The signs are ring-shaped, red, scaly or blistery patches forming on the skin. Without knowing it we all come into frequent contact with the spores – or seeds – of the fungi that cause ringworm, either as they float about in the air or as we touch others who have them – but remarkably few of us become infected.

It's also remarkable that with ringworm – like athlete's foot, which is caused by the same family of fungi – several members of the same household can share a bathroom, or even a bed, without catching the disease. Nobody knows quite why, although we do know that we all vary considerably in our susceptibility to most diseases.

Before the introduction of effective anti-fungal medicines over the past fifty years, ringworm used to be a real scourge often causing a person's hair to fall out, leaving the scalp covered in unpleasant sores. In the old days drastic measures, like a course of x-rays, were taken to try to 'sterilise' the skin. However, such x-rays had disastrous results in later years – they certainly cured the ringworm but, with hindsight, it was like using a sledgehammer to crack a nut, since the powerful x-ray could cause growths to appear on the affected skin many years afterwards.

Nowadays, following your doctor's recommended course of treatment is probably the best advice for curing ringworm. With today's effective anti-fungal preparations (on prescription or from a pharmacy), the skin will eventually clear. However, if you remain in conditions that encourage the fungus to grow, then it can return, even when anti-fungal preparations have been taken. Once the anti-fungal effect wears off the fungus may return anyway, regardless of the conditions you are in, although after each treated attack this becomes much less likely as the body gradually builds up a resistance.

Thrush

So many women suffer from thrush without knowing there are a variety of ways to prevent and treat it. Thrush is a common vaginal infection due to the multiplication of a yeast-like fungus known as Candida albicans, which occurs naturally in the vagina, mouth and digestive tract. When the body's natural balance is upset, perhaps by pregnancy, diabetes, antibiotics, sexual contact with someone who has the condition or even having a period, the fungus can multiply and cause great irritation and discomfort.

The most common symptoms are soreness, itching

and occasionally swelling of the vagina and vulva. There is also often a whitish, curd-like discharge which looks a bit like cottage cheese and has no smell. Often there is a burning feeling at the entrance to the vagina. Sometimes, too, your partner may carry the organism on his penis and develop an itchy rash. If he does, he should be treated as well.

There are a number of misconceptions about thrush. It hasn't been scientifically proved that the contraceptive pill causes the condition and it is quite likely that women who are on the pill are getting recurrent attacks because their partners are not using a barrier method of contraception, particularly the sheath – the man could be harbouring the thrush under his foreskin, reinfecting his partner every time they make love. This is why it is important for the male partner to be treated at the same time as the woman. All he has to do is rub the cream under the foreskin and around the tip of the penis.

Thrush isn't a venereal disease – it *can* be sexually transmitted, but virgins have been known to get it. This is because the fungus produces lighter-than-air spores which, should they happen to land on a warm, moist place on the body, may develop into thrush, especially if that person's defences are low for some reason.

Thrush can be very depressing for the sufferer, but if the rules are followed it is treatable. Many women suffer numerous attacks – and once it has been diagnosed by a doctor it can easily be recognised by the sufferer. However, if you experience thrush for the first time, or if you are in any doubt about the condition, always seek the advice of your doctor.

Two new safe and effective over-the-counter medicines for the treatment of vaginal thrush, called Femeron and Canesten, are now available from pharmacies. Your doctor may prescribe another form of anti-fungal cream or pessaries, or capsules containing itraconazole (an anti-fungal agent).

There are some very simple things that a woman

should do to guard against further attacks. Make sure you wash every day. When you go to the loo, it's particularly important after a bowel movement to wipe yourself from front to back (not from back to front), just as you would to avoid cystitis. And don't use perfumed soaps, deodorants, bubble baths, etc, which could cause irritation. Some women have found that using tampons or an intrauterine contraceptive device has put them more at risk of developing the condition. Others have found that wearing synthetic underwear or tight-fitting trousers helps the fungi to thrive because of the warm, moist environment.

Some women have told me that they believe tampons irritate the vagina because of the chemicals within them. However, tampons nowadays don't contain irritant chemicals. Instead, I believe it is the mere physical presence of the tampons that causes the increased irritation.

Vaginal douches should not be used, although some women do seem to find relief when they insert fresh, live natural yoghurt into the vagina. This contains 'healthy' germs – the lactobacilli – which compete with and may overcome the thrush-causing micro-organisms. I'm a great believer in this simple and natural remedy.

Thrush can sometimes occur under the breasts, and may affect babies orally and in the nappy area.

Finally, the nails can also be infected by a skin fungus. This is particularly difficult to treat since the tough nail plate itself is not supplied with blood and is almost impermeable to liquids. So neither the body's antibodies nor antibiotics can penetrate the nail to destroy the fungus.

HEAD LICE AND PUBIC LICE

Head lice and pubic lice can cause severe itching. Once you get them they won't let go until you do something about them! Head lice are tiny brown insects with six short, stubbly legs. They're about the size of a pin-head and live on human scalps, laying six to eight eggs a day of a creamy-brown colour. They turn white when the baby louse, called a nymph, has hatched. The remaining pearly white husk is commonly known as a nit, and at this stage is a harmless shell.

The eggs are attached near the base of the hair shaft – a favourite spot is around the ears. Each louse takes two weeks to mature and lives for twenty to thirty days if undetected. The lice feed on blood, using their specially developed mouth-parts to pierce the scalp. They even inject a local anaesthetic into the scalp to prevent their host feeling any pain, and an anticoagulant to stop the blood clotting, thus making it easier for them to feed! They can eventually make your head feel very itchy and worse – hence the well-known phrase 'I feel lousy'! This is because, after about 10,000 bites, your immune system becomes understandably irritated.

To check whether someone has head lice, dampen the hair and then bend the head over a plain sheet of paper. Comb thoroughly to see whether any insects drop out. Then quickly part the hair to look out for moving lice. A magnifying glass will help. You can also see the nits attached to the hair shaft.

Head lice can sometimes be a problem among schoolchildren because with them the head louse has never had it so good. We and our children are healthier and cleaner than we have ever been, and the head louse loves it. Clean, healthy heads provide it with the perfect environment. Head lice can't jump or fly, nor do they live in bedding, furniture or clothes. The only way they can be passed on is by close head contact – a single louse can visit several heads in one day just by walking from one to another.

So if you or your children have head lice, please don't worry or feel ashamed about going to see your doctor. In the UK more than a million people a year get head lice, so there's no point being embarrassed about it. It's also pretty well impossible to prevent children catching lice from each other. Like chicken pox, it's just another one of those things children are likely to catch once they start mixing with others.

Pubic lice (commonly called crabs) are mostly passed on during sexual intercourse. Irritation and itching in the pubic region can be extremely uncomfortable and intense. The lice can often be seen at a glance and look like tiny scabs. Your GP can prescribe one of a variety of lotions and shampoos and you can also buy them without a prescription from your pharmacist. Some, such as one containing carbaryl (Carylderm) or malathion (Derbac-M), will also be suitable for getting rid of head lice.

When applying a shampoo or lotion, remember to ensure that no part of the scalp or pubic hair is left uncovered; pay particular attention to the nape of the neck and behind the ears when dealing with head lice. There are three main insecticides in use that destroy head lice and their eggs – carbaryl, pyrethroids (phenothrin, permethrin) and malathion. They are all equally effective if used according to the directions. But health authorities change their recommendations for louse treatment preparations every two to three years to prevent the lice building up a resistance to them.

Bear in mind, too, that should a member of your family have lice, you should treat everyone – parents, grandparents, even lodgers – and then check them once a week to ensure they're still clear. This applies equally to pubic lice since these can be passed on by older children who share a bed or if they regularly get into the beds of other family members. However, the main way in which pubic lice are passed on is by a regular bed partner, especially one who is in intimate contact. Make sure your children's friends don't have lice either or there could be a risk of re-infection. It's wise – if not essential – to inform your child's school if you discover head lice.

Then, after treatment, encourage all your family to comb their hair thoroughly every day, since the female louse – and there are many more of them than the male – must cling on to two hairs to survive; as combing or brushing separates the hair, the louse will die and fall off harmlessly. It also breaks the lice's legs making them drop off the hair.

ICHTHYOSIS

In ichthyosis the skin tends to become rough and take on the appearance of fish scales ('ichthus' is, in fact, the Greek word for fish). The skin is extremely dry, and becomes hard and cracked. There's no doubt that some forms of this skin problem are inherited.

See under 'Dry skin' (pages 68–9) for advice on how to cope.

INTERTRIGO

Intertrigo is an inflammation of large moist skin surfaces that are in close contact. These areas become red and painful. The condition is most common in babies (in the skin creases of the groin), the elderly (in women, for example, under pendulous breasts) and the obese (where an 'apron' of abdomen becomes so large that it hangs down). Your doctor may prescribe an ointment containing a mild topical steroid, such as hydrocortisone, to reduce inflammation and help heal the infected area, or one combined with an anti-bacterial or anti-fungal agent. But to make sure the problem doesn't recur it is important to maintain good standards of hygiene.

KERATOSES

Keratoses, also called senile warts, seborrhoeic warts and keratoids by American doctors, are regrettably common in middle and later years. These lumpy freckles are unsightly but do not necessarily, or even usually, develop into skin cancer. However you are better off without them. Sufferers often describe them as greasy and they are frequently crumbly on the top – indeed, the top layers will often flake off and then be replaced. No one knows precisely why they appear or why some people get them more than others (see 'Warts' on pages 98–9).

LENTIGO (OR SENILE LENTIGO)

With this condition, which usually affects the elderly, a dark spot will appear on the person's skin – often on the cheek. This will enlarge over the years and part of it may turn malignant although, fortunately, it is usually of a very low order. A mark that is causing concern can be removed, although a very elderly person may not want that to happen. Usually, a specialist will be content to leave it alone in the knowledge that it is not likely to be the main health problem.

LICHEN PLANUS

This skin problem – an itchy 'rash' of raised spots that are purple in colour – isn't all that common. The name is given to the usually flat, slightly round, slightly purplish eruptions because they look a little like lichen plants. The spots usually appear on the front of the wrists and forearms and sometimes the trunk and the lower legs. It can also affect the mucous membranes inside the mouth and the anus. No one knows what causes it.

Some people suffer from it much more than others. It may cause an itch which comes and goes and varies from mild to severe. Anti-inflammatory creams can keep the condition at bay and it will often disappear on its own.

LINEA NEGRA

Pregnant women are sometimes concerned about changes to their skin, particularly when they develop a brown line straight down the tummy from just below the naval to the pubic hair. This is nothing to worry about. The line is called the linea negra and is due to increased pigmentation produced by melanin cells during pregnancy. (Moles, birthmarks and freckles also tend to get darker at this time, as does the belly button.) The line starts to develop at the fourteenth week of pregnancy and is most noticeable in brunettes, less so in fair-haired women and often absent altogether in red-heads. It is not in any way harmful.

The pigmentation cannot be washed away but will begin to fade soon after delivery. However, it can take a few months to disappear completely and the belly button occasionally remains discoloured for several years.

MILIA

These are also called epidermal cysts. They are very small and cause the skin's surface to feel rough. They are due to accumulations of hard layers of cells near the surface of the skin, called horn cells. No one knows why they arise. The larger ones can be gently shelled out.

(They are not to be confused with miliaria which are also of pin-head size and arise after excessive heat. The everyday name for milaria is 'prickly heat', which is described on page 81.)

MOLES

What's the difference between a freckle and a mole? Well, I'll explain. In young people, freckles and moles are very similar if looked at under a microscope. To the naked eye, a freckle is usually a flat brown blemish and a mole is a raised brown one. Both are technically called a naevus, due to the naevoid cells in the skin from which they appear. Though these cells will have been present from birth, a visible blemish may not appear until years later. If visible at birth, they're called birthmarks (see pages 61–3).

MYXOEDEMA

This affects the skin, but it is not specifically a skin condition. It's due to an underactive thyroid (hypothyroidism) and seems to be more common in women than men, usually after the age of forty-five. It is a fairly common condition and develops slowly as a result of the deficiency of the thyroid hormone leading to a lack of energy, weight gain, dry lifeless hair, a deeper, croaking voice and a thickening and yellow tingeing of the skin. The sufferer will also usually also be anaemic.

No one knows why the thyroid starts to underfunction, though it is likely to be due to a degenerative change which comes with age in the majority of cases. Treatment consists of taking a daily 'replacement' of thyroxine in tablet form.

PHEMPHOID AND PHEMPHIGUS

These are relatively uncommon conditions of the skin which cause large water blisters. Both are likely to be due to the body's defences over-reacting and so attacking the skin – known as an auto-immune condition. Steroids are the usual treatment.

PITYRIASIS ROSEA

This is an inflammatory red rash which usually starts in just one place – known as the 'herald' patch because it tells you that other patches will follow, usually after about nine or ten days. When the rash appears on the rest of the trunk, the individual patches, which are usually oval-shaped, can vary in size – they can be almost as small as a pin-head or as large as a 50 pence piece. They result in itching which can be relieved with Calamine lotion. No one knows what causes them. The rash will usually go after six to eight weeks.

The condition tends mostly to affect those aged between ten and thirty. Again, no one knows why, though it's probably due to a virus infection that is being met for the first time.

PRICKLY HEAT

Prickly heat is an extremely irritating skin rash which develops in hot weather. It occurs – in some more than others – when the small blood vessels under the skin widen as the temperature rises. The extra blood supplied to the surface acts as the body's radiator, allowing heat to escape. This blood supplies the extra liquid which the sweat glands release as sweat. As the tissues swell with blood and tissue fluids, the skin becomes congested and the pores are squeezed and then blocked. The sweat builds up under the skin and causes a rash known as prickly heat or Miliaria rubra.

Sufferers from prickly heat will witness the emergence of tiny red pimples or blisters – the tissues look red because the small blood vessels are open wide, while the engorged tissues cause discomfort, the prickly feeling.

There's no quick simple remedy for this condition, but if you can immerse yourself in water to keep cool, you should feel better. Covering yourself with light, white clothing will help and, obviously, keeping out of direct sunlight is a good idea, too. Calamine cream or lotions will cool the skin and antihistamine tablets can bring great relief.

SCABIES

Scabies is another problem that can cause much discomfort. Itch mites, technically known as sarcoptes scabei, can cause intense irritation to the skin (and the owner!) when the female mite burrows down to lay her eggs. It's a condition that's spread by direct contact between children, sexual partners and often throughout a family home. Try not to scratch too much as this can lead to the skin becoming infected, making the condition even more unpleasant. When a person has developed scabies they can feel quite disgusted at the thought of insects living in their skin!

If you sleep in the same bed as someone who has scabies or wear their clothes you allow the mite to have easy access to more territory – *your body*. Like an army, they dig themselves in, causing irritation and the need to scratch. In fact they can make us itch all over even though they are only infecting one particular area.

Nevertheless treatment is straightforward, using scabicidal drugs which kill the mites. Applying benzyl benzoate emulsion; Asabiol, Quellada or Tetmosol usually do the trick. But it's essential to wash all your clothes and bedding to make sure no mites remain.

SKIN CANCER

Skin cancer develops in three main ways. The most common form is the rodent ulcer, medically known as a basal cell carcinoma. A rodent ulcer is so called because it invades locally – literally gnawing away at the skin and its underlying tissues. If it is not treated by removal, x-rays or freezing, it can gnaw into deeper tissues such as bone. In the majority of cases, a rodent ulcer can be completely cured. So, if you have a pimple or tiny sore which persists or which worries you, it should be examined by your doctor, especially if it arises on those parts most exposed to the sun, such as face and hands.

Malignant melanomas are not so common, although estimates suggest that in the UK in the past ten years, as more of us holiday abroad, their occurrence has doubled. A malignant melanoma arises when the melanin-producing cells in the skin run riot. Warning signs include a mole changing appearance, becoming swollen or itching, bleeding, weeping or crusting over, in addition to having a reddish edge. Also look out for any existing or new mole which has a ragged, rather than curved outline.

Since on average we have perhaps thirty moles on our body, we mustn't get overly worried that these are automatically going to turn nasty. It's important to remember that almost one in two malignant melanomas arise in previously clear skin. This puts the problem into perspective since obviously all white-skinned races have far more clear skin than they have skin pigmented by a mole.

Although sunburning, and even suntanning, is the main reason for a malignant melanoma developing, the sun is also more commonly responsible for rodent ulcers. For instance, in Australia – a very sunny country in which white-skinned races have only lived for the last two hundred years – both MM and rodent ulcers are much more common than in Britain where there's far less sun.

One more point about MM: while the sun is largely responsible it doesn't just act directly. That is to say, the melanoma doesn't just arrive where the sunburn occurred. Hot sun on the skin as a whole diminishes the body's defences, which is why cold sores break out on lips in the sun. This overall effect is also why MMs can develop on areas of the body which have had less than their fair share of the harmful exposure.

So the message is clear. Holidays are for rest and relaxation – for these alone you will return home feeling and looking better. Seeking a deep suntan while on your summer holiday will soon be as unfashionable as smoking heavily in a crowded room. By protecting yourself from the direct rays of the sun, with light airy clothes and a sun hat, your skin will still lose its pasty white winter colour because the sun's rays are reflected off sea, sand and buildings.

The third type of skin cancer is called squamous cell carcinomas. These are also uncommon. They are generally more malignant than the rodent ulcers, and can grow and be transported elsewhere to form secondary cancers. Consequently, doctors will always recommend that they are treated without delay. They may appear first as a hard nodule with a warty surface or as a sore, usually painless, which won't heal but which bleeds very easily and spreads quite rapidly. It may take on the appearance of a small cauliflower or have raised edges which tend to curl outwards. Surgical removal or x-rays are usually the recommended treatments.

SKIN TAGS

Are skin tags a cause for concern? Or are they best left alone? Well, let me tell you what they are.

Skin tags are small growths of skin most commonly occurring on the neck, groin, armpits or trunk. They are usually no more than 5 mm long and are wider at their top than at their base. Nobody really knows why they appear – you might just be one of those people who are more susceptible to them than others. However, they do seem to affect women more than men.

If they're not in an unsightly place or don't get in the way most doctors will suggest that they are left alone. Your GP may snip them off with a sterile pair of scissors and then put pressure on the point of removal until it stops bleeding. If you don't fancy this, he can give you an injection of local anaesthetic first, although the process is rarely very painful. Alternatively, some doctors will suggest that a clean piece of white cotton is tied around the base of the tag, pulled comfortably tight and then left there. Under these conditions the tag will usually drop off in a day or two and shouldn't bleed. In any case, before you do anything, it's best to seek your doctor's advice.

STRETCH MARKS

Pregnant women often worry about the possibility of stretch marks and ask me how they can avoid them. Answer – you can't. Some women don't get them at all and others get a lot. Those who are overweight to start with are usually worst affected, but this is by no means always the case.

Stretch marks also arise in growing teenagers, in the heavily overweight and in sufferers of Cushing's Syndrome, when the adrenal glands are over-working.

No one knows what causes them and apart from masking them with cosmetics, not much can be done to improve their appearance.

SUNBURN

As I've explained elsewhere, a minimum amount of sunshine on the skin is beneficial – it supplies vitamin D and helps to keep the more harmful germs that live on the skin at bay – but there is no longer any doubt that continuous and prolonged exposure to the sun or a sunbed's rays can, in fact, be harmful to white people.

This harm is observed in all sorts of ways. The skin usually ages prematurely, with wrinkling and dark brown blemishes, which are often accompanied by an ugly thickening of the top skin layers (called solar keratosis). Skin changes that we notice as we get older – wrinkles and loss of elasticity – are now believed to be due mainly to damage from the sun. About 70 per cent of this skin damage, which may take years to show, probably occurs in childhood as a young child's skin is thinner than that of an adult and more likely to burn.

Quite apart from these cosmetic disadvantages, there is also no doubt that deep tanning on holiday, even for only two weeks a year, enormously increases the risks of developing a skin cancer. At best this will be a basal cell cancer, otherwise known as a rodent ulcer; at worst it can cause a malignant melanoma (see pages 83–4).

Sunburn is no different to any other burn. The skin will flake or fall off as soon as the underlayer is ready, and if you pick it off too soon, you will be pulling away the tender underskin that is forming, causing it to bleed (and also causing the developing tan to look rather patchy and unattractive). Of course it is great to be in a warm, sunny climate – swimming, sitting under a sun shade or partaking in water sports – provided we keep covered with light but protective clothing.

For those parts that we do intend, or can't avoid, exposing to the sun, then good, powerfully protective sunscreens are readily available. But, having applied them, you still shouldn't take any chances with the sun. Remember, too, that babies and young children are particularly vulnerable to the harmful rays of sun, so always use a sun protection cream designed for their delicate skins. Babies under six months old should be kept out of the sun anyway, not just because of the risk of sunburn, but also because of heatstroke which can be even more dangerous.

Avoiding the sun between 11 a.m. and 4 p.m. – when

ultra-violet radiation is at its most intense as the sun is directly overhead – may not necessarily be the best safeguard as times vary according to geography and seasonal changes. So a good tip is to watch your shadow: when it's the same height as you are, the sun's rays are at an angle of 45 degrees and therefore less dangerous – provided, of course, that you use an adequate sunscreen. If your shadow is shorter, you're more likely to burn.

If you do suffer from sunburn, the painful effects usually only last for a few days, followed by itching as the skin heals. Lotions containing calamine or aloe vera, with perhaps menthol, phenol or camphor, have a cooling effect on the skin. Blisters should not be burst and you should drink plenty of water just in case you have become dehydrated. If the skin is burnt or peeling, stay out of the sun until it has healed completely. If symptoms are severe, always consult a doctor.

SUN ALLERGY

Sun allergy, or polymorphic light eruption (PLE), is triggered by the skin reacting unusually to the sun's ultraviolet rays, resulting in a red, itchy rash which sometimes turns into small watery blisters. Dermatologists tell us that PLE is most commonly triggered by the ultraviolet A (UVA) component of sunlight. Sunlight also produces ultraviolet B (UVB) and visible light. Although UVB rays are far stronger than UVA (UVB being the major cause of sunburn, skin ageing and skin cancer) the actual amount of UVA reaching the earth's surface at midday during the summer is said to be one hundred times greater than UVB.

PLE is yet another indication that too much exposure to sunlight is not good for our health. The vast majority of people who have this condition are able to control it by avoiding prolonged exposure to the sun, and applying high-protection sunscreens.

URTICARIA

More often known as hives or nettle rash, urticaria is a very common skin condition, affecting one in five people at some time in their lives. Women are particularly prone, perhaps because of hormonal influences.

With 'ordinary' urticaria, weals – intensely itchy raised marks on the surface of the skin – suddenly develop. They are usually short-lived, lasting for a few hours or days, although they can last longer. They can be any size, appear anywhere on the sufferer's body and may be numerous. They are usually pale in the middle and red around the edges and are due to dilation of the capillaries – small blood vessels under the skin – which makes their walls more permeable and enables clear fluid, called serum, to leak out. If enough serum leaks out, blisters may form.

So what causes this reaction in the blood vessels? Often it is due to an increased circulation of histamine, a chemical normally present in the body. This increase can be triggered by many factors, including various foods, drugs and inhalants such as pollens, house dust and animal 'dander' (skin flakes which the animal sheds naturally plus various chemicals its body gives off). Foods that are frequently responsible are shellfish, strawberries, eggs, nuts, chocolate, tomatoes, pork, milk and yeast. Artificial colourings and preservatives can produce the reaction, too.

Aspirin can also cause, or aggravate, urticaria. Penicillin is another possible culprit, as are the non-steroidal anti-inflammatory drugs often prescribed for arthritis. Sometimes contact with certain substances will bring the symptoms on – cosmetics are one example. Insect stings can also cause this type of reaction, which may even be life-threatening if the breathing is affected.

Urticaria sufferers whose attacks occur in response to triggers such as these are often, but not always, allergy-prone individuals – from hay fever, asthma or eczema, for example – and the tendency can run in families. Anxiety may also play a part.

Other constituents in the body – called catecho-lamines – can, by irritating the tissues surrounding them, have the same effect on the blood vessels as hist-amine, and almost anything can act as the trigger.

Most cases of urticaria tend to resolve themselves in due course, and in the meantime antihistamine tablets prescribed by your doctor usually relieve the symptoms. For mild cases, soothing creams containing antihista-mine (which stop the effects of histamine on the blood vessels beneath the skin) or creams and lotions contain-ing calamine help calm down any swelling and itching by cooling the skin, especially if these preparations con-tain menthol, phenol or camphor.

VIRAL SKIN PROBLEMS

Chicken pox and shingles

Chicken pox, a common childhood virus, results in watery blisters appearing on the skin, causing intense itching. You'll notice it developing when a rash of small red spots appears on the body and then spreads to the arms, legs, face and head. The spots change to watery blisters that either burst or shrivel up and crust over. The virus can make you feel generally unwell and there may be a raised temperature.

I'm often asked whether it's true that it is more un-pleasant if you develop chicken pox as an adult. It most certainly is. However, sometimes a person can have chicken pox without realising it, as one can have what is known as a 'subclinical' attack in which no spots appear. Nine out of ten people will have chicken pox at some time as it's very infectious.

Calamine lotion will help ease the itching, and paracetamol suspension can make children feel less uncomfortable. A medicine such as Periactin (cyproheptadine hydrochloride) may be prescribed which blocks the action of histamine. It can soothe itching and gently sedate the sufferer. Other antihistamine medicines supplied by your pharmacist may also bring relief.

Shingles is a rash of blisters on the skin accompanied by a severe stinging pain, caused by the virus which is also responsible for chicken pox. You cannot catch it directly. If you do contract the virus from someone with shingles (by rubbing yourself against the rash) you will develop chicken pox. This is because shingles is the manifestation of the Herpes Zoster virus that has been sitting in certain nerve cells in the body since the time you had chicken pox.

Antibodies to the virus develop in the bloodstream during the chicken pox infection (to prevent further attacks), but the virus is able to settle and lie dormant in a non-infectious state in the 'junction boxes' of nerves. Often it will cause no further trouble, but if it does, the result will be shingles.

All manner of events can trigger an attack. If you're emotionally or physically exhausted, or suffering from illness or injury – indeed, if your body's defences are not at their best for whatever reason – the virus can become active. The older you get, the more likely you are to develop shingles – of those who reach eighty-five, at least one in two will have suffered from it, and the older you are the more severe it tends to be.

The first symptom is usually pain over the area of skin supplied by the nerves harbouring the virus. The most common place is down the side of the body, along a line following a rib. It can occur on both sides of the chest, but it is an old wives' tale that if it meets in the middle the outcome is fatal – that just isn't true.

To have the best chance of success, any treatment should be given early on, preferably at the painful stage which can be when (or just before) the blisters appear, and should certainly be given within forty-eight hours of their appearance.

Your doctor can prescribe a course of anti-viral tablets or applications which may help to lessen and/or shorten the attack. Anaesthetic ointments or over-the-counter medication containing calamine can also be soothing.

The surrounding skin should be kept clean to prevent other germs from infecting the blisters, as this could interfere with healing and lead to scarring. Antibiotics may be needed if infection does occur.

Cold sores and herpes

Cold sores appear as little blisters which develop into weeping sores. They usually grow in groups around the lips but may also occur on other parts of the face. If precautions are not taken, the virus responsible can also be spread to other people, or to other parts of the body – the eye, for example – with potentially more serious results.

I'm often asked if you are born with the virus that causes cold sores. The answer is no, you have to come into contact with it. Cold sores are caused by the herpes simplex type I virus, of the herpes group, others of which cause chicken pox, shingles and glandular fever. A slightly different strain of the same virus, known as type II, is the one usually responsible for outbreaks of herpes blisters around the genital area, although type I may be the culprit here, too.

The herpes simplex type I virus is very common indeed – it's being passed around most of the time and is responsible, for example, for many if not most sore throats. Once the HSVI has entered the body, usually via the throat, it is carried around in the bloodstream and frequently establishes itself in a certain part of a nerve near the throat. It rests there until our defences are low, when it breaks out, travelling down the nerve to the lip or nose, causing the cold sore on the surface. It also inflames the nerve itself, and as this nerve carries sensations to the brain the sufferer often feels pain.

It is estimated that about half the adults in this country are carriers of type I herpes. Most will have had their first, often symptomless and undetected, infection in early childhood. Many will never have another attack, and some may have one after an interval of several years. A small percentage will have recurrent episodes every few months.

Various factors can contribute to the reactivation of the virus – exposure to sunlight, an infection or being generally 'run down', for example. For a woman, an outbreak of cold sores is more likely to occur during menstruation. However, with each new outbreak, the body produces further antibodies which accumulate to fight the virus. This means that, in time, outbreaks tend to lessen in both frequency and severity.

For severe outbreaks there are effective drugs available – the anti-viral drugs acyclovir (Zovirax now also available over the counter) and idoxuridine (Herpid, Virudox). Treatment with Zovirax should begin as early as possible after the onset of an infection. Cold sores are highly contagious while the blisters are present and as the virus is also found in the saliva of the sufferer save your kisses until the blisters have gone.

You can infect vulnerable parts of your own body, via the fingers, if you touch the sores and do not wash your hands afterwards. Any area of broken skin is especially susceptible and it is particularly important not to touch the blisters and then rub your eyes, as the virus may be transferred and cause an ulcer on the delicate membrane covering the eye. If this is not diagnosed and treated soon enough, it can damage the sight.

Mothers with cold sores should take extra care and wash their hands frequently, and always after applying medication – babies and toddlers are extremely vulnerable to cold sores as they won't have had time to build up their antibodies. It is also important to keep the flannels, towels, eating and drinking utensils of the sufferer separate from those of the rest of the family.

Many sufferers of recurrent cold sores notice definite warning symptoms before an outbreak – for instance, a 'prickly' feeling in the area of skin usually affected. If you apply an anti-viral ointment or solution during this phase, you can shorten the duration of the outbreak considerably, and during the first attack it may even quell it sufficiently to prevent further outbreaks.

A simple old wives' remedy is to apply fresh, cold coffee to the area on a piece of clean cottonwool every two or three hours, allowing it to dry. This may sound primitive, but it does seem to work for many people, so it is worth trying if a doctor or pharmacist isn't available. Other than this, the sores should just be kept clean and dry.

A regular, well-balanced diet will help maintain your general health and may therefore prevent attacks. Also be sure to use a good sun-blocking cream applied liberally to the lips before and during a concentrated period of sunbathing. There is no cure for cold sores, so if you are prone to them, keep a supply of your favourite remedy handy so that you can start the treatment when the warning symptoms first occur. Eventually you will develop your own natural resistance and the cold sores should become a thing of the past.

Genital herpes is transferred from one infected person to another during sexual intercourse. Just like a cold sore on the lips, there is no magical cure. This makes it sound very frightening, but fortunately complications (such as infections of the urethra and deeper tissues) are very rare and only occur as part of an initial attack. Inconvenient and distressing though herpes may be, it is rarely a life-threatening disease.

After an attack, the virus lies dormant (or 'nests') in the nerves of the genital area. Then, when the body's immune system is below par, the infection can erupt again. So it's important to obtain treatment as soon as herpes is suspected in order to minimise the symptoms. The most effective drug available to do this is acyclovir (Zovirax) in cream or tablet form, which helps the body's own defences fight the virus. Another anti-viral drug used to treat herpes is inosine pranobex (Imunovir).

If you suffer from herpes, take reassurance from the fact that attacks become less and less frequent with every year that passes. Many people suffer only one attack while others have to put up with it for years. But most report that it stops as suddenly as it starts.

It's essential for any man or woman who has genital herpes to insist on using a condom during sex, especially if they suspect an attack is coming on. If possible they should avoid sex altogether during this time. There is no cast-iron guarantee, the passing on of herpes between attacks is unlikely, but I would advise herpes sufferers to use condoms even when symptoms aren't present.

With both types of herpes, close physical contact is required for infection of others to occur, so if reasonable precautions are taken during the week or so that the blisters last, there should be little cause for concern.

On occasions I have been asked whether people with atopic eczema have lower resistance to some viral infections, such as cold sores. The symptoms do seem to be more severe for them but I'm not sure why. The likely reason is the inflammation caused by the eczema.

With a highly contagious condition such as impetigo or herpes, you need to be very thorough to prevent infection. Pillow cases, towels and face flannels should not be shared and you should boil them once they have been used. Also, you must not touch infected areas of skin (unless of course to put on medication).

WARTS AND ALL

Quite simply, warts are small, dry lumps of skin often seen on the hands, knees and face. They develop when a virus invades the skin cells and causes them to multiply very quickly. There is more than one virus – called a papilloma virus – that causes warts. They're spread through contact with skin that's been shed from a wart, or by the virus coming into contact with damaged skin, particularly if it is warm and moist. That's why it's advisable to use only your own towels until your warts have cleared, to reduce the risk of spreading the condition to other members of your household.

Sometimes, warts just appear out of the blue and the sufferer is unable to remember having come into contact with anyone who has them. Magically, it seems, they can disappear just as quickly.

There are all sorts of old wives' tales for conjuring the warts away. If you hear of one, and it's harmless – like rubbing your warts with stones which have to be wrapped up and left at the crossroads on the way to church for another unsuspecting person to pick up and acquire your warts – what have you got to lose? And I don't believe the person who picks the stone up is likely to suffer one jot either! If the wart goes away, I won't spoil things for you by saying it was due to disappear anyway. But, the fact is, warts of this kind more often than not clear up on their own.

Warts are a nuisance as they can be so ugly, but they're usually harmless. They tend to last longer on adults than they do on children, so if your child's wart doesn't cause any discomfort, is not too unsightly and doesn't get in the way, it's best to leave it alone until it clears up of its own accord. That way, you won't run the risk of scarring if it's removed.

For adults, warts can be removed using solutions or creams which usually contain a caustic such as strong acetic acid that will destroy any tissue it's applied to (so protect the surrounding skin), or a keratolytic drug such as salicylic acid that will soften and loosen the wart. These treatments can be obtained from pharmacies. Other methods of removing warts are similar to the treatment for verrucas (see pages 97–8).

Genital warts

Women can develop genital warts in or around the vagina or on the cervix, and men can have them on the penis. These warts are due to a viral infection, usually transmitted during sexual intercourse, although they may occur for other reasons.

Most genital warts develop from a root-like base below the surface of the skin and each has its own blood supply, so this must be taken into account when dealing with them.

Never treat any warts on the genitals or around the anus with over-the-counter remedies. Go to your own doctor or to a sexually transmitted disease clinic. There, a definite diagnosis will be made and you will be checked for other infections that are often contracted at the same time. The wart will generally be treated with a 'paint', which contains podophillin, a caustic solution that destroys the wart and the virus within it. You will often be instructed how to apply this yourself, or be assigned a local nurse who will do it for you.

Molluscum contagiosum

Despite the exotic-sounding name, this is a common childhood viral infection. Again, children with eczema may suffer more than others. The infection manifests itself on the skin as clusters of small bumps which resemble warts. When looked at closely, many will have a small crater at the top. The sites usually affected include the face and body.

These bumps do clear up on their own, though they may take many months. They can also be treated individually by a doctor or at the skin clinic, by removing the contents of the spots and applying a drying up solution.

Verrucas

Verruca normally occur on the sole of the foot, but are just the same as a wart elsewhere on the body. Because of their location they get pressed inwards and appear flat, and are usually moist. The skin surface is rough and the shape irregular. They often have tiny black centres, appear in groups and become painful if they press on a nerve.

Verrucas are caused by a virus entering the foot, possibly via a slight area of damage – as is the case with common warts – and are very infectious, particularly among children. The virus loves warmth and moisture – and soggy feet! – so is easily passed on in such places as swimming pools and showers. If you have verrucas, therefore, you shouldn't go barefoot until they have cleared up. Many swimming pools now provide plastic socks for children with verrucas so that they do not infect others.

Yet verrucas are a mystery. Some people can walk through moist, damp, undoubtedly contaminated places and never get one, and no one knows why!

Feelings run high on the subject of verrucas. Mothers, schoolteachers, and even chiropodists, believe that 'sufferers' should be removed from contact with others and write strong letters to the 'authorities' stating that children with verrucas must be kept out of swimming pools. But many doctors and specialists – me included! – maintain that this segregation makes not one iota of difference to the spread of the virus. The debate continues.

Verrucas can be treated with over-the-counter remedies which usually contain a keratolytic – salicylic acid, for example – to soften the verruca so that it can be cut out or pulled off. If possible, cover the verruca with a ring-pad plaster to protect the surrounding skin. Put a small quantity of the ointment or paint on the verruca, then cover it with a plaster for two to three days. After several applications, the verruca should separate from the surrounding healthy tissue. If this doesn't happen within about two weeks, consult your doctor or chiropodist.

After a few days of treatment, the verruca will probably appear white or blanched. This is perfectly normal and indicates that the treatment is working well.

Other methods for removing verrucas if they become painful are cryotherapy, 'freezing' them with liquid nitrogen; 'burning' with an electric cautery; or scraping them out with a scalpel, called a curette. Often a local anaesthetic will be given first to numb the surrounding area.

If you suffer from recurrent or persistent verrucas you should consult a chiropodist, and diabetics should always see their doctor about foot problems because they can more easily pick up infections.

Seborrhoeic warts

'Is it true that warts are not always due to a virus?' I have often been asked. The answer is yes. Some non-viral, wart-like brown or black eruptions are the so-called 'seborrhoeic' or senile warts which many people develop on their body, temple or scalp as they get older. Although they can look very similar to viral warts, they are usually darker in colour.

They are caused by the changes that come with age – as well as the effects of the sun – as opposed to a virus. They don't often cause problems, but they can sometimes itch severely. It's best to have them examined by a doctor who may advise having them removed. As these seborrhoeic warts can enlarge or change colour, they can worry the sufferer, who will wonder, quite justifiably, whether it is developing into a cancerous growth. Because the true diagnosis may not be immediately obvious – even sometimes to a skin specialist – removal will often be advised, just to be on the safe side.

In general, it's advisable to let a doctor examine any wart when it first appears and especially, as with moles, if it changes in size or colour, or begins to bleed or itch. But usually warts remain nothing but an annoying blemish.

6: HOW TO HANDLE YOUR DOCTOR

Many people with skin problems do feel aggrieved by us doctors. One psoriasis sufferer told me that many GPs seem to write you a prescription for a steroid cream before you've even sat down, without bothering to ask you the extent of the problem and how you are feeling psychologically.

Maxine Whitton, who spoke about her vitiligo on pages 54–6, believes that skin problems don't feature that highly in a GP's training.

> GPs themselves are a big problem for people with skin conditions. Dermatology is not a very big part of their training. It can sometimes just be a week or two – that's pathetic. So I believe that we're done at the first hurdle. With vitiligo, for instance, GPs tend not to know very much about it and because there is no really effective treatment they say you just have to live with it. But people need information about the problem, particularly if it's spreading. It's very discouraging for a sufferer to encounter that sort of approach. One doctor once told me that there was nothing he could do for me and that there was no point referring me to a dermatologist because I would just take up room in the clinic! A lot of people can shrivel up at that sort of response, which just compounds the problem.

I'm often asked whether it's worth bothering a doctor, especially if the symptoms turn out to be the result of something inconsequential. But if you are worried about something *you should always check it out*. As most people don't have any medical training, the only practical criterion you can apply when deciding whether or not to go to the doctor is your own unease and worry — so let this worry be your guide.

Your doctor can then either recommend investigation or treatment for worrying new symptoms, or reassure you that there's nothing to be concerned about. Such reassurance is part of a doctor's job, a part that will save you — and him or her — time in the long run.

And a note here for anyone who does not like their GP or would prefer a different one. You are perfectly entitled to change. In fact, you can change your doctor without even giving a reason — it's that uncomplicated. Go along to the practice of your choice, preferably with your medical card, and ask whether or not you can be put on their list.

I do understand how some people find it hard to keep faith with the medical profession when they feel they haven't received much sympathy or haven't been listened to. But remember, doctors aren't mind-readers and you are the only person who can explain how you are feeling and how badly you want to be helped.

You may say your doctor never listens to you, but perhaps he could equally say that you never talk to him. No matter how busy your GP may seem, it's still important to make the most of the time you have with him. So there's absolutely no harm in preparing yourself mentally for a visit, or taking in a list of points you want to raise, in case you feel nervous or rushed once you're inside the surgery or if you're worried you'll forget to mention one of your symptoms or fears.

I know it's an easy thing to say, but don't allow yourself to be intimidated by medical staff. If you don't understand what you're being told, make sure you ask for it to be explained more slowly or more simply. You needn't feel embarrassed or stupid. You certainly won't be the first person who's had difficulty grasping all the facts. And you won't be the last, either.

If you're worried about something in particular,

make sure you ask questions about it. Very often some reassurance is all you need.

While we're talking about doctors, I'd like to say a few words about the medicines prescribed for skin conditions. Always follow you doctor's or pharmacist's instructions on how often and how much you should use. Don't think that if the treatment isn't working it's because you're not using enough. Twice the amount of medication won't necessarily mean twice the desired effect. If the treatment isn't working, discuss it with your doctor.

And when your doctor hands you a prescription with your name on the top, it is meant for you and *you alone*.

7: COMPLEMENTARY TREATMENT

Most practitioners of unconventional therapies prefer the use of the term 'complementary' medicine rather than 'alternative' because they feel their treatment should work side by side with more conventional methods.

ACUPUNCTURE

For many people acupuncture gives rise to images of human pin-cushions, with needles stuck in here, there and everywhere. In reality, it has been an accepted form of treatment in China for around five thousand years, and these days more and more people in the West are turning to it for a wide assortment of ills. Many people believe it is extremely effective in easing a variety of conditions, by – in simple terms – stimulating the patient's own healing responses. Conditions that can be helped include skin problems, headaches and migraine, back pain, tinnitus, insomnia and even depression.

So what does acupuncture involve and how can it help you? One theory is that it works by stimulating the brain to produce the body's natural painkillers, the chemical endorphins – raised levels have been detected in tests twenty minutes after treatment. Traditional acupuncture is a 'holistic' form of medicine – a philosophy which not only treats the symptom but aims to improve the total well-being of the patient. Practitioners believe that many physical conditions are worsened by, or even a result of, emotional stress, poor diet, and other factors. So your first visit to an acupuncturist will probably include detailed questions about your lifestyle and a thorough examination. The tongue is especially important in making a diagnosis so don't be surprised if this comes under careful scrutiny.

Acupuncture aims to correct any disharmony between what practitioners call the body's Yin and Yang. An imbalance, they say, leads to disease. There are different traditions of acupuncture but all revolve around the principle that the body has an intricate network of pathways, 'meridians', which carry vital 'energies' through the body. These cannot be seen but can be detected using special techniques and can be likened – albeit loosely – to the nerve pathways known to Western doctors.

There are twelve main meridians either side of the body, each related to specific organs, such as the heart, liver and stomach. Twelve different pulses on the wrists also relate to the various organs. When the traditional acupuncturist is deciding on treatment these pulses will be measured and many factors taken into consideration.

Each meridian has points along it in precise positions, called 'acupoints'. Very fine needles are inserted into several of these points depending on the problem. By inserting needles or by using pressure, it is claimed, the correct flow and balance of energies can be restored. The needles are solid and finer than those for injections and you normally feel only a slight prick as each is inserted.

Some practitioners – many GPs, for example – have undertaken a short course in acupuncture (not involving the whole philosophy) and will use it in a limited way, for example, to relieve pain. Often acupuncture can be used in conjunction with conventional medicine to improve the patient's general health. Always be sure to go to a well-qualified acupuncturist – those with letters after their name such as BAAR or TAS. Any adverse effects should then be most unlikely and you can be confident that the needles used will be properly sterilised.

ALEXANDER TECHNIQUE

The Alexander Technique is a gentle method aimed at relaxing muscles and improving posture by undoing bad sitting and standing habits. The technique was first developed in the 1890s by Frederick Matthias Alexander, an Austrian actor and reciter. Having become hoarse during performances, he worked out a new approach to balance, posture, and movement which resulted in a great improvement in his general health.

His technique is a gentle one which relaxes muscles by teaching the pupil to sit, stand and move gracefully without causing any strain. In this way, so the theory goes, you can rid yourself of the persistent tension that so often causes a variety of problems, particularly headaches, backache, tiredness and depression. Many dance and drama schools teach the technique and it's even becoming popular in sport – the 1990 World Cup Italian football team is said to have used it in training.

The instructor will teach you to listen to your body and help you find ways to change your posture to avoid using unnecessary effort and to stop you slipping back into your old habits of slouching or hunching your shoulders. Many people push out their jaw and stretch their neck when getting up from a sitting position, instead they should use their leg muscles to push themselves up. Other bad habits can be drawing your chin towards your chest or rounding your shoulders. The technique helps you understand when you are working against your natural poise and allowing your bad habits to take over.

An Alexander Technique teacher will point out to you tension you weren't even aware of and how you trigger off this tension at the thought of movement. He will then instruct you on how to prevent this.

It's very difficult to get across in words exactly how the technique works so if you are interested in it it is worth trying a lesson or two to understand what all the fuss is about. Some people find one lesson so relaxing they want to learn more about the technique in order to adapt its teachings into their everyday life.

The Alexander Technique is taught on a one-to-one basis because the teacher needs to place his or her hands on the pupil's body as he or she explains the method. Also, different people have different bad habits so treatment needs to be designed to your individual lifestyle. The teacher usually chooses a simple movement, say sitting or standing, to work on. Some time is also spent lying on a table while you are taught how to perfect the technique.

It's beneficial to begin with two or three lessons a week, gradually spacing them out as you acquire the ability to practise on your own. You can discuss alternatives with the teacher if this is impractical. If it does appeal to you, it's generally accepted that you'll need a course of twenty to thirty lessons. Some local authority education centres run group classes. The cost of a lesson is comparable to a session with an osteopath, acupuncturist or other alternative therapist and some teachers will offer an introductory lesson free of charge. Teachers will have completed an intensive three-year course approved by the international STAT organisation (Society of Teachers of the Alexander Technique).

AROMATHERAPY

Aromatherapy is said to be relaxing and, as such, a good way to treat stress and build up a resistance to it. It's also a good way of indulging yourself and allowing time just for you.

The process involves the use of powerful, natural plant essences derived from flowers, leaves, stems, roots or bark, used in massage or added to your bath water. The oils can also be inhaled by adding a few drops to a bowl of hot water. You can either consult a professional aromatherapist or buy essential oils from health shops, pharmacists and the Body Shop. Nelson & Russell make a range of essential oils – for example, their Ylang Ylang and Orange Bath and Massage Oils are said to be good for resting and relaxing, as are the Body Shop's Rose or Lavender. Lavender, in particular, helps relieve tension-related problems, and lavender oil is also thought to be useful for soothing skin conditions such as eczema and psoriasis.

But a word of warning – neat essential oils shouldn't be used directly on the skin but should be diluted in a 'carrier' oil. And some aromatherapy oils should not be used if you are pregnant or suffer from epilepsy or certain other conditions. Don't leave the tops off containers either, as the oils are highly volatile and can soon evaporate. Keep them well away from children and never use them near your eyes. Do not take them internally either.

HERBALISM

Herbs seem to get into everything these days! Of course, they have always added flavour to cooking, and herbal teas such as camomile and peppermint have long been popular. Now, bath oils, shampoos, face and body lotions containing a variety of herbs sell like hot cakes as we are encouraged to believe that all things natural are good for us.

'Herbs' (which include a variety of plants, flowers and even trees) have been used for thousands of years to cure or prevent disease and even today 85 per cent of the world's population is largely dependent on herbal medicine. For a long time no one really understood how or why herbal treatments worked, but more recently scientists have been able to separate many of the active chemical ingredients from the healing plants and set up tests to observe their effects.

Some of these substances are now produced synthetically in laboratories and form the basis of modern drugs. For example, digoxin (a heart stimulant) is the synthetic, pure form of the active ingredient of digitalis, found in foxgloves. And salicylates, derived from the willow bark, is now produced synthetically as aspirin. However, herbalists believe that by using only the main, active ingredient of the plant, one is losing the benefits provided by the other ingredients which are all working in harmony. Therefore they always use the whole plant.

Because of shortage of funds and other difficulties, there have been very few scientific trials using the whole plant (although some research has now proved that feverfew can be effective against migraine). This lack of conclusive evidence is one reason why doctors are sceptical of herbal medicine. Nevertheless, herbal treatments are subject to official scrutiny, and licensed herbal products will have satisfied the Government's Licensing Authority in respect of safety, quality and efficacy. GPs can prescribe such products on the NHS if they consider them to be in their patient's interest and if they know enough about herbal medicine to feel competent about prescribing them.

Herbalists believe that medicines derived from the whole plant work in a similar way to food, for example providing essential vitamins and minerals – which help protect the body against illness – and enzymes which aid absorption of food. Some plants have within them a natural antidote to the side-effects a medicinal ingredient could cause if it were extracted and given in isolation. For instance, ephedrine – a drug often prescribed by doctors to relieve bronchial symptoms – comes from the plant Ephedra sineca and can cause an increase in blood pressure. But in fact the plant itself includes an ingredient that keeps blood pressure down. Herbalists can point to many such instances where the ingredients in the plant counterbalance each other.

Herbal medicine aims not just to treat a particular

symptom, but to improve the overall physical and mental well-being of the patient. Diagnosis and treatment will include advice on diet and lifestyle, as these may be partly responsible for the symptoms. In fact, herbalism takes so many factors into account that two people with apparently identical symptoms may be given quite different prescriptions. Professional herbalists are trained to use many of the same diagnostic methods as doctors and to refer people for x-rays and other specialist investigations or treatment, if necessary.

Medicines are usually given in the form of a 'tincture' – a concentrated solution made from herbs which have been soaked in water and alcohol. Sometimes the herbalist provides the actual plants from which to make an 'infusion' (similar to tea) or a 'decoction', whereby the plants are gently simmered for some time and the juices then strained off. Medicinal herbs can also be given as suppositories, ointments and poultices.

It is part of a medical herbalist's training to learn the most effective quantities that must be used of each plant, but the constituents of the plant can vary, depending on such factors as where it is grown and the time of year it is picked. This means that it is impossible to measure accurate dosages, and is another reason why most orthodox doctors still have their doubts about herbal medicine.

The herbal remedies available from pharmacies, health food shops and supermarkets may be helpful for minor problems. Examples skin problems include Gerard House Blue Flag Root Compound for minor acne and eczema, Heath & Heather Skin Tablets, a traditional remedy for spots, skin blemishes and dry eczema, Nelsons Graphites Cream for dermatitis, Nelsons Calendula Cream for sore and rough skin, or Nelsons Evening Primrose skin cream to soothe dry skin. Potters have a range of preparations, ointments and others, for example Psorasolv for psoriasis and Eczema ointment.

But, if symptoms are persistent or become severe,

consult a registered medical herbalist for a full assessment and tailor-made prescription. Look for the initials MNIMF or FNIMH after the practitioner's name to avoid quacks – a professional herbalist will have done four years' training.

Most herbal remedies are mild enough for children, and even the names of many healing plants sound soothing – lemon balm, comfrey, meadowsweet and speedwell, for instance. However, like anything else, they can be harmful if used incorrectly or taken in excess. Recently a man died from drinking far too much carrot juice – so always follow the instructions carefully.

Some conventional and herbal medicines work well together but others can interact badly, so always tell your GP and herbalist about any medication you are taking.

HOMOEOPATHY

Homoeopathy is said to be a completely safe form of therapy and homoeopathic medicines are available under the National Health Service.

This form of treatment is relatively new in comparison with acupuncture. It was first developed around two hundred years ago by a German physician, scholar and chemist, Samuel Hahnemann, from the principle that 'like cures like'. Symptoms are treated by administering a minute dose of a substance which if given in larger quantities to a healthy person will actually *cause* those symptoms. (This principle is sometimes used in conventional medicine also – for instance, controlled doses of radiation are given to cure cancer, though excessive doses can actually cause the problem.)

Homoeopaths believe in the body's natural ability to heal itself. A homoeopath will therefore aim to give a remedy which will encourage the process of stimulating the body's natural forces of recovery. This is unlike a conventional doctor, who prescribes medicines to suppress symptoms (aspirin, for instance, to bring down a temperature, or antihistamines to dry up a runny nose).

Many homoeopaths are qualified doctors who have done a further year's training in homoeopathy. They may become GPs or work in homoeopathic hospitals (there are about six of these in the UK), their treatment is available on the NHS, or they may consult privately. If you do consult a homoeopath who is not also a doctor, make sure he or she had undergone full homoeopathic training at an approved college.

Homoeopathic remedies said to be useful for dry skin conditions include *Graphites*, *Rhus. Tox.* and *Sulphur*.

OSTEOPATHY

I've included this therapy because a person's general well-being is so often enhanced by responsible, hands-on treatments.

The General Council and Register of Osteopaths describes the treatment as the 'science of human mechanics' as it is concerned with the structural and mechanical problems of the body. Osteopaths are keen to point out that the therapy is more than manipulation alone. They use a variety of techniques from soft-tissue massages, to stretching, as well as the high-velocity thrust that most people associate with the therapy. This type of manipulation is a minor part of the treatment and some osteopaths rarely, if ever, use it.

Osteopathic treatment tends to be pleasant and relaxing and tailored to suit the needs of the individual concerned. That's why when you first visit an osteopath you will be thoroughly questioned about your medical history and when the symptoms first began.

The osteopath may also give you advice on posture, diet, your lifestyle, or stress, particularly if any of these factors seem to aggravate or trigger your skin problem.

Don't entrust yourself to an osteopath without first checking his or her qualifications. You can always phone the Osteopathic Information Service on 071 439 7177.

REFLEXOLOGY

The origins of reflexology can be traced back thousands of years and the technique is thought to have been used by the Ancient Egyptians. The art of foot reflexology today was established in the 1930s by an American therapist called Eunice Ingham. Some people believe that this method of treatment can be helpful in alleviating all manner of ailments, from bunions, headaches, insomnia, to vertigo, even high cholesterol and deafness. I have to admit, I'm not entirely convinced it can work for many of these conditions though I would support their 'cure' for headaches, for example, and I know that some psoriasis sufferers find reflexology a useful means of controlling stress.

Reflexology works on the understanding that there are areas, called reflex points, on the feet and also hands, that match up with each organ, gland and structure of the body – the sole of the foot is thought to represent a map of the body. The four arches of the spine – cervical, thoracic, lumbar and sacral – are reflected in the four arches of the feet.

A treatment of reflexology can last around thirty to forty minutes and is likely to involve a variety of massage techniques using the thumb and index finger plus a rotation of the foot called reflex rotation or pivot-point technique. The technique is a gentle one and many people find it quite pleasurable. It's considered that the main benefit is its powers of relaxation, which can relieve stress and tension. It's also said to improve blood supply and to encourage the unblocking of nerve impulses.

*

I am in favour of alternative treatments – but do let both your doctor and the complementary practitioner know that you're seeking the help of them both. And listen to their advice and their opinions on the value or the dangers.

Remember that these treatments may help but I don't believe they can always *cure* a skin problem. Also be aware that you don't have to have your doctor's approval to try these treatments, although, as I've said, I would suggest checking with him first to rule out any possibility of risk in your individual case.

It seems that many psoriasis sufferers are driven to try complementary treatments out of sheer frustration. And it's thought that acupuncture may be able to help some cases. Eczema sufferers have found that alternative treatments such as homoeopathy, herbalism (particularly Chinese herbal medicine), osteopathy and naturopathy have helped relieve symptoms. Remember, though, that eczema has no cure and that atopic eczema can clear up on its own but then return just as suddenly.

As for vitiligo, the Vitiligo Society believes that reports of success with homoeopathy, herbalism and acupuncture are anecdotal rather than based on hard evidence. The Society's advice to sufferers is that it's up to the individual to decide whether to embark on a course of alternative medicine. Certainly try to establish the likely cost of such a treatment before embarking on it.

Some people with skin problems turn to alternative treatments because they believe that conventional treatment doesn't really work for them. Sally, a twenty-five-year-old computer technician, has suffered from eczema to varying degrees since she was a baby.

For more than twenty years I have had a mixture of steroid creams, from mild to strong. Then, when I was about twenty, I developed marks, not unlike stretch marks, on the inside of my thighs where my skin has thinned. The skin there is also puckered. It makes me very self-conscious, particularly when I go swimming. It's a memory of my treatment with steroid creams that isn't going to go away. Doctors still try to give me steroid creams, but if I had known what effect they would have had on my skin I would never have used them in the first place.

For the past few months I have tried Mora therapy which apparently is quite well known in Europe. It has a holistic approach since my skin is a reflection of my whole body. It's like electroacupuncture and you're also treated with homoeopathic medicines. I haven't had eczema for three months. I still have very dry and red skin but it's such a relief not to have the itching all the time. I am also careful to use lots of moisturiser on my skin and I use lots of emollients in my bath. I drink lots of water each day. I'm careful about my diet now. I avoid dairy products, citrus fruits and tomatoes. I find that if I eat any of these things I have an upset stomach and my skin will flare up in a few days and then get very itchy.

I really think that it's worth giving an alternative treatment a try. It may not be suitable for everyone but I was concerned about the damage the other medicines were doing to my skin – so from that aspect alone I believed it was worthwhile.

HELPFUL ADDRESSES

UNITED KINGDOM

Acne Support Group, PO Box 230, Hayes, Middlesex UB4 9HW.
A counselling and self-help group. If you'd like to join, write enclosing an SAE.

British Homoeopathic Association, 27a Devonshire Street, London W1N 1RJ. Tel: 071 935 2163.
For books, advice, information and a list of practitioners.

Council for Acupuncture, 179 Gloucester Place, London NW1 6DX. Tel: 071 724 5756.
Send £2.50 and an A5 addressed envelope for a directory of British acupuncturists.

General Council and Register of Osteopaths, 56 London Street, Reading, Berkshire RG1 4SQ. Tel: 0734 576585
For addresses of registered osteopaths in your area.

Institute for Complementary Medicine, PO Box 194, London SE16 1QZ. Tel: 071 237 5165.
Send a large SAE with three loose stamps and a clear indication of what kind of information you'd like. The institute holds the British register of complementary practitioners and can give advice on training courses.

National Eczema Society, 4 Tavistock Place, London WC1H 9RA. Tel: 071 388 4097.
The society was set up to support, educate, inform and raise money for research. For details of the society's wide

range of literature, plus the quarterly journal *Exchange*, and for information on membership, send a large SAE.

The National Institute of Medical Herbalists, 9 Palace Gate, Exeter, Devon EX1 1JA. Tel: 0392 426022.
Contact the institute for a list of practitioners.

The Psoriasis Association, 7 Milton Street, Northampton, NN2 7JG. Tel: 0604 711129.
The association is a self-help group, providing social contact, advice and collecting funds, which aims to help people affected by psoriasis by changing attitudes and improving awareness through its programme of research, education and support.

The Red Cross Beauty Care and Cosmetic Camouflage Service, 3 Grosvenor Crescent, London SW1X 7EJ. Tel: 071 235 5454.

The Vitiligo Society, 97 Avenue Road, Beckenham, Kent BR3 4RX. Tel: 081 776 7022.
The society offers support to vitiligo sufferers and their families either by letter or phone. It also has a growing network of locally based support groups. Members receive a regular newsletter with information on the latest research. An information pack is available covering aspects of the problem, such as protection from sunburn and details of cosmetic camouflage techniques.

AUSTRALIA

Eczema/Dermatitis Association of South Australia, PO Box 331, St Mary's 5042

Psoriasis Association, Suite 11, Second Floor, 119 Leichhardt Street, 4000 Brisbane. Tel: (07) 832-4524.

Psoriasis Association of NSW, c/o Skin and Cancer Foundation, 376 Victoria Street, Darlinghurst, NSW 2010.

CANADA

The Canadian Psoriasis Foundation, National Office, Suite 500A, 1306 Wellington Street, Ottawa, Ontario, K1Y 3BZ. Tel: (613) 728-4000.

INDEX